Transplant Protocol

이식 프로토콜
매뉴얼

삼성서울병원 이식외과

MANUAL

 SAMSUNG MEDICAL CENTER

이식 프로토콜 매뉴얼

1판 1쇄 인쇄	2020년 2월 19일
1판 1쇄 발행	2020년 2월 28일
1판 2쇄 발행	2021년 1월 22일

지 은 이	삼성서울병원 이식외과
발 행 인	장주연
출 판 기 획	김도성
책 임 편 집	안경희
편 집 디 자 인	정다운
표 지 디 자 인	김재욱
일 러 스 트	메디컬일러스트 그리닥
발 행 처	군자출판사
	등록 제4-139호(1991. 6. 24)
	본사 (10881) 파주출판단지 경기도 파주시 회동길 338(서패동 474-1)
	전화 (031) 943-1888 팩스 (031) 955-9545
	홈페이지 | www.koonja.co.kr

머리말

삼성서울병원은 1995년 신장이식 1996년 간이식을 시작한 이래로 지금까지 5000예에 육박하는 신장이식 간이식 췌장이식을 진행해 왔습니다. 한국 이식의 역사와 마찬가지로 초기에는 선진국이라고 불리는 나라의 자료를 하나씩 배워 왔고, 작은 배움 하나 하나를 모아 지금의 프로토콜을 이룰 수 있었습니다. 지금은 국내외의 많은 기관에서 삼성의 수술과 프로토콜을 배워가고 있습니다. 이러한 성과를 이룰 수 있었던 것은 20년의 시간 동안 우리의 이식 프로그램이 자리 잡도록 헌신해주었던 많은 전임의, 전공의 선생님들과 코디네이터를 포함한 여러 간호사 분들이 계셨기 때문입니다. 이 곳을 통해 고마움을 전합니다.

이 책은 교과서가 아닙니다.

이 책을 세상에 내 보내면서 많은 고민과 논의가 있었습니다. 대부분은 과학적 근거에 기반한 내용이지만, 일부 내용은 단지 경험에 기반하여 수립된 부분도 있습니다. 경험주의자들의 결과물이라는 비판도 있을 수 있겠지만, 그 작은 경험 하나 하나는 한 생명을 잃지 않기 위한 우리의 노력이라는 점도 잊지 말아 주십시오. 작게는 우리 병원에서 장기이식을 진행하면서, 궁금한 부분을 해결하는데 도움을 되길 바라고, 조금 넓게는 임상 현장에서 환자를 진료할 때, 그리고 새로운 곳에서 이식 프로그램을 만들어 가는 분들께 작은 도움이 되기를 희망합니다. 또한 우리의 첫걸음이 우리 보다 앞선 사람들에게 하나하나 배워서 이것을

머리말

이루어 왔듯이 이 책의 작은 한 부분이라도 이식을 하고 있는 다른 선생님들께 도움이 되기를 희망합니다.

우리나라의 장기이식이 세계 최고의 임상 성적과 연구 성적을 보여준다는 것은 부정할 수 없는 사실이 되어버렸습니다. 지금의 자리에 있기까지 수없이 많은 의료인의 희생과 노력이 있었고, 10년동안 10배 가까이 증가한 뇌사 기증자의 수가 보여주는 것처럼, 수많은 사람들이 타인의 목숨을 살리기 위해 기꺼이 장기를 기증해 주셨습니다. 또한 자신과 가족의 목숨을 구하기 위해 많은 환자와 가족들이 자신의 생명을 맡겨 주셨기에 가능한 일이었습니다. 기증자와 환자분들에게 고개 숙여 감사의 마음을 전합니다.

마지막으로 많은 일러스트레이션 작업을 진행해 준 유진수 교수와 김미승 연구원에게 지면을 통해 고마움을 전합니다.

2021년 봄을 기다리며
삼성서울병원 이식외과 교수 조재원

집필진

조재원 (삼성서울병원 이식외과)   박재범 (삼성서울병원 이식외과)

최규성 (삼성서울병원 이식외과)   김종만 (삼성서울병원 이식외과)

이교원 (삼성서울병원 이식외과)   유진수 (삼성서울병원 이식외과)

도움 주신 분

김갑수 (삼성서울병원 마취통증의학과)   백경란 (삼성서울병원 감염내과)

신동현 (삼성서울병원 소화기내과)   이상훈 (삼성서울병원 소아외과)

길은미 (삼성서울병원 중환자의학과)   허경민 (삼성서울병원 감염내과)

고재훈 (삼성서울병원 감염내과)   김상진 (삼성서울병원 이식외과)

김경덕 (삼성서울병원 이식외과)   이옥주 (삼성서울병원 이식외과)

권지은 (삼성서울병원 이식외과)   양재훈 (삼성서울병원 이식외과)

임마누엘 (삼성서울병원 이식외과)   정은성 (삼성서울병원 이식외과)

김복녀 (삼성서울병원 장기이식센터)   홍승희 (삼성서울병원 장기이식센터)

이윤미 (삼성서울병원 장기이식센터)   강은진 (삼성서울병원 장기이식센터)

백선미 (삼성서울병원 장기이식센터)   김현정 (삼성서울병원 이식외과)

차소라 (삼성서울병원 장기이식센터)   오시영 (삼성서울병원 장기이식센터)

일러스트 제작

메디컬일러스트 그리닥 (유진수 김미승)

CONTENTS

CHAPTER 01.

TRANSPLANTATION IMMUNOLOGY

I. Main characters of transplantation immunology

1. T-lymphocyte

골수에서 형성되어 thymus에서 negative selection (self에 강한 affinity
를 갖는 cell을 제거) 및 positive selection (self를 인식하지 못하는 cell
을 제거)을 거쳐 CD8+ T-cell, CD4+ T-cell, regulatory T-cell로 분화
된다. CD8+ T-cell은 cytotoxic T-cell로 주로 작용하며, CD4+ T-cell
은 immune response를 증폭시키는 helper T-cell로 주로 작용한다.
Regulatory T-cell은 immune response를 조절하는데, 주로 억제하는 역
할을 한다.

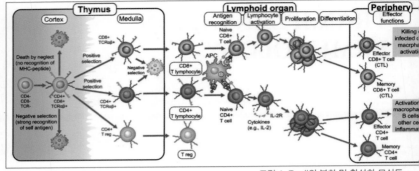

그림 1. T-cell의 분화 및 활성화 모식도

2. B-lymphocyte

골수에서 형성되어 CD4+ helper T-cell 또는 다른 자극에 의하여 활성화
되면 plasma cell로 분화하여 antibody를 분비하게 된다. 활성화된 B-cell
중 일부는 memory cell로 분화하여 spleen 또는 lymph node에 존재하
며, 재차 노출되는 자극에 강한 면역반응을 유도하게 된다.

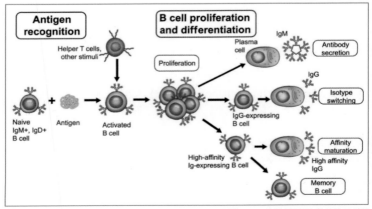

그림 2. B-cell 의 분화 및 활성화 모식도

3. Antigen presenting cells (APC)

1) Dendritic cell은 가장 강력한 antigen presenting cell이며, co-stimulatory molecule과 함께 antigen을 제시하여 naïve T-cell을 activation시킨다.

2) B-cell과 macrophage도 APC의 역할을 할 수 있으나, 이미 활성화된 effector T-cell에만 작용할 수 있다.

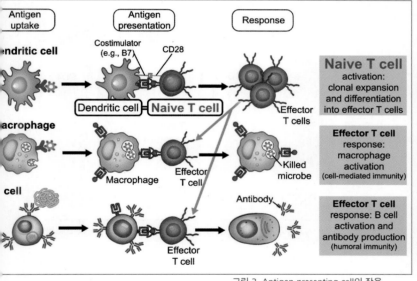

그림 3. Antigen presenting cell의 작용

4. Major histocompatibility complex (MHC)

가변성이 매우 높은 유전자로부터 발현된 peptide binding molecule로 T-cell에 의하여 인식되는데, class I과 II가 있으며 "이름표"라고 생각하면

된다. Class I은 nucleated cell의 대부분에서 발현되는 반면, class II는 APC에서 주로 발현되고, 여러 자극에 의하여 활성화된 신장 세포에서도 발현되는 것으로 알려져 있다.

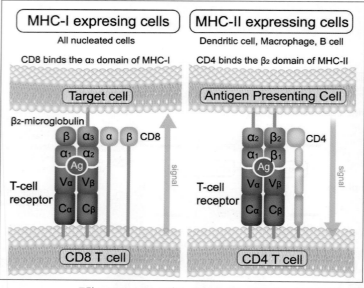

그림 4. MHC molecule과 T-cell의 interaction 및 MHC molecule 발현 세포

5. Complement system

Antibody가 세포를 공격하는 기전 중 하나로, 보체계(complement system)가 활성화되면 결국 세포막에 구멍을 내는 membrane attack complex (MAC)을 형성하여 세포사멸이 유도된다. Complement 활성화 과정 중 세포막 표면에 C4d라는 부산물이 남게 된다.

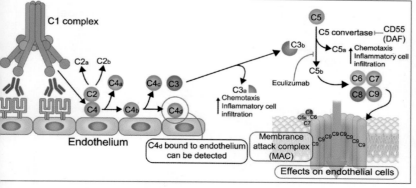

그림 5. Complement system activation 과정

II. Basic immune response

1. Antigen presentation

어떠한 경로를 통해서든 antigen이 들어오거나 체내에서 생성되는 경우 APC에게 그 antigen이 흡수되고 내부 processing을 거쳐 MHC molecule 위에 얹혀진 상태로 APC의 표면에 표출된다. APC는 Lymph node (LN)나 spleen과 같은 secondary lymphoid organ으로 이동하여 T-cell에게 antigen을 제시하게 된다.

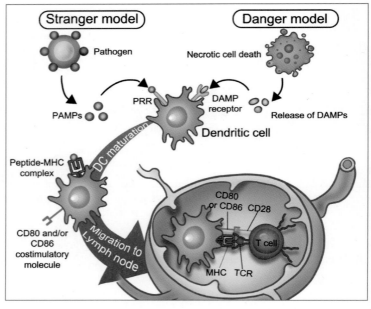

그림 6. Antigen presenting cell이 antigen을 T-cell에게 제시하는 과정

2. Secondary signal and MHC restriction

APC에 의하여 제시된 antigen을 T-cell이 인식하고 활성화되기 위해서는 두 가지 조건이 만족되어야 하는데, 첫째, 본인(self)의 MHC molecule에 antigen 이 제시되어야 하며(그림 7), 둘째, co-stimulatory secondary signal의 자극 이 동반되어야 한다(그림 8). 이 두 조건이 만족되지 않으면 T-cell은 활성화되 지 않는다. 이러한 co-stimulatory signal 중에 가장 대표적인 것은 B7-CD28 pathway 이며 APC표면의 B7과 T-cell의 CD28이 결합하여 stimulatory signal을 형성한다.

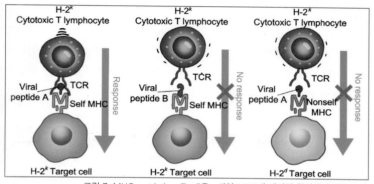

그림 7. MHC restriction, T-cell은 self의 MHC에 제시된 항원에만 반응한다.

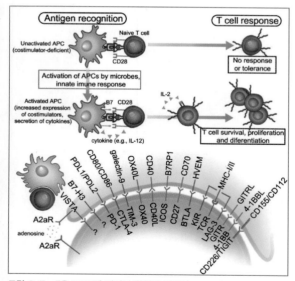

그림 8. T-cell은 MHC에 제시된 항원과 더불어 secondary co-stimulatory signal이 같이 동반되어야 반응한다, 이중 가장 대표적인 것은 B7-CD28 pathway이지만 현재 수많은 secondary signal이 밝혀져 있다. (초록색은 stimulatory, 빨강색은 inhibitory second signal)

3. T-cell activation

Lymphoid organ에서 위에서 설명한 일련의 과정을 거쳐 T-cell이 자극되면, T-cell은 IL-2를 분비하여 스스로를 더욱더 활성화시키고 분열하게 만든다. 대부분은 활성화되어 effector T-cell로 작용하며, 일부는 memory T-cell이 되어 재차 자극이 되는 경우 강한 면역반응을 유도한다.

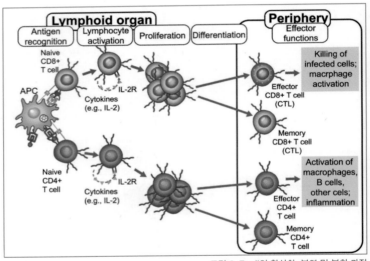

그림 9. T-cell의 활성화, 분열 및 분화 과정

4. B-cell activation and antigen producing

B-cell은 LN 또는 spleen의 germinal center에서 APC와 CD4+ helper T-cell의 자극을 받아 활성화되며, 분열하고 분화하여 결국 antibody를 생성하는 plasma cell이 된다. 일부는 memory B-cell이 되어 재차 자극이 되는 경우 강한 면역반응을 유도한다.

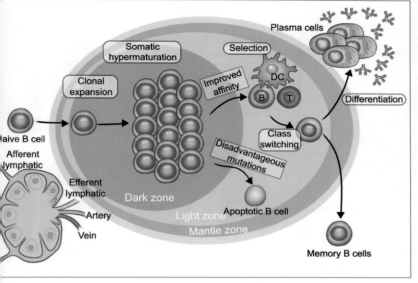

그림 10. B-cell의 활성화, 분열 및 분화 과정

5. Action of antibody

1) 항체(antibody)는 다양한 mechanism으로 면역반응을 유도하는데 직접 항체를 중화시키기도 하고, 탐식작용을 유도하고, 항체 유도 세포사(antibody dependent cellular cytotoxicity, ADCC)를 유도하기도 한다.

2) Complement activation 을 통한 면역반응을 유도하기도 하는데, 항체와 C1이 결합하면서 이 반응이 진행된다(세부 내용은 그림 5. 참조).

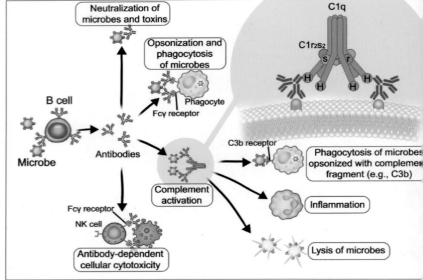

그림 11. Antibody에 의한 면역반응의 mechanism

III. Immune response after transplantation

장기 이식 이후에 일어나는 일련의 면역반응은 아래의 〈그림12〉와 같이 일어나며 APC가 이식편의 antigen을 T-cell에 제시하고, T-cell이 그러한 antigen을 인식하게 되는 (1) allo-antigen recognition과 활성화된 T-cell이 이식편에서 면역반응을 유발하는 (2) rejection과정으로 나누어 볼 수 있다.

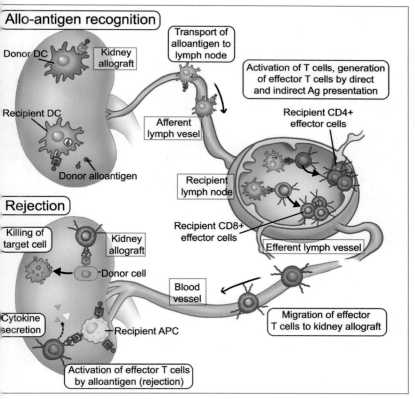

그림 12. Immune response after transplantation의 전반적인 개요

1. Allo-antigen recognition

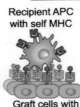

그림 13. Allo-antigen recognition의 mechanism

1) Direct recognition

Donor의 APC가 donor의 MHC에 donor의 antigen을 제시하고 이를 recipient T-cell이 인지하는 과정이다. 이식 초기의 강력한 면역반응의 원인이 된다. 하지만, 이 과정은 〈그림7〉에서 설명하였던 MHC restriction (self의 MHC가 아니면 인식하지 못하는 현상)에 위배되는 현상이다. 이러한 현상이 일어나는 이유는 〈그림14〉와 같다. Antigen과 MHC molecule의 복합체가 self의 MHC와 유사한 모양을 갖게 되는 현상으로 인하여 non-self 의 MHC를 인식하게 된다.

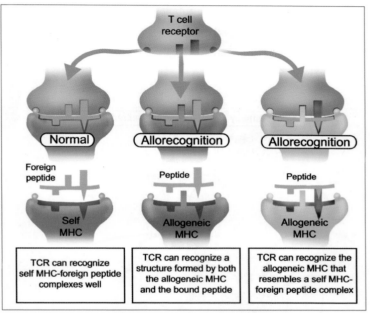

그림 14. Non-self MHC와 antigen의 복합체가 allo-recognition을 유도하는 mechanism

2) Indirect recognition

Recipient의 APC가 recipient (self)의 MHC에 donor의 antigen을 제
시하고 이를 recipient T-cell이 인지하는 과정이다. 이는 일반적인
antigen presentation 과정과 동일한 과정이며, 이식 후 거부반응이 발
생하는 일반적인 mechanism이다.

2. Rejection

1) T-cell mediated rejection

- Direct 또는 Indirect recognition 과정으로 활성화된 CD8+

cytotoxic T-cell이 renal tubule, parenchyma, 그리고 vascular endothelium을 공격하는 과정이다. 결국 활성화된 T-cell은 B-cell을 활성화시키고 antibody의 형성 및 antibody mediated rejection으로 진행될 수 있다.

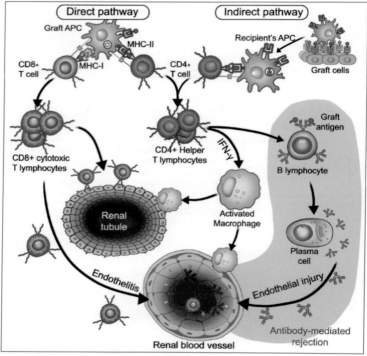

그림 15. T-cell mediated rejection 의 과정, antibody mediated rejection으로 진행될 수 있다

2) Antibody mediated rejection

(1) Hyper-acute rejection

이식 전 이미 recipient의 체내에 존재하는(pre-formed), 기증자 특이적인(donor-specific) antibody가 있는 경우, 즉각적인 면역반응이 발생하며 결국 혈액응고작용으로 진행되고 미세혈관의 혈전이 형성된다.

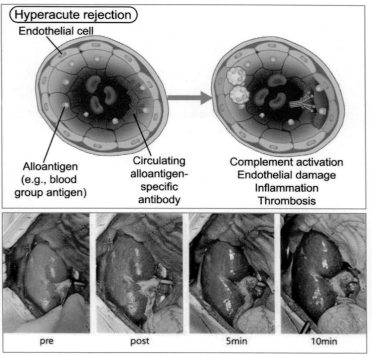

그림16. Hyperacute rejection 의 mechanism과 xeno kidney transplantation 이후 hyperacute rejection이 발생한 kidney의 macroscopic appearance

2) Donor specific antibody

주로 donor의 MHC에 대한 recipient의 antibody를 donor specific antibody (DSA)라고 한다. 이식 전에 이미 있는 경우(pre-formed) 와 이식 후 새로이 발생하는 경우(de novo)로 나누어 볼 수 있으며, pre-formed DSA는 hyperacute rejection을 유발할 수 있으므로 탈감작 (desensitization)이 필요하다. 이식 후 여러가지 원인에 의하여 graft 의 조직으로부터 지속적으로 antigen이 생성되고 APC에 의하여 processing되어 T-cell로 전달된다. 이러한 과정을 거치면서 recipient의 B-cell이 donor의 MHC에 대한 Ab를 형성하게 되는데 이렇게 만들어지는 DSA를 de novo DSA라고 할 수 있다. 이러한 de novo DSA는 〈그림 17〉 과 같은 여러가지 작용을 하게 되고, 그 결과 antibody mediated rejection을 일으킨다. 그 중 complement system을 활성화 시키는 작용도 하게 되고, 그 결과 endothelium에 C4d 라는 부산물이 남게 된다. (그림5. 참조) 따라서, C4d염색이 AMR의 진단 기준이 된다.

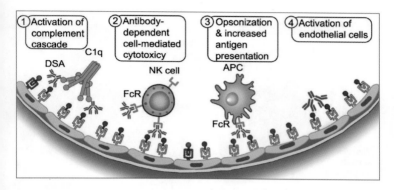

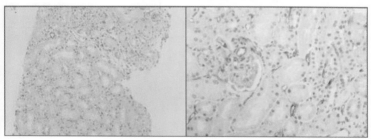

그림17. De novo DSA가 allograft에서 antibody mediated rejection을 유도하는 mechanism과 kidney allograft의 AMR에서 C4d deposition

3) Chronic rejection

- Chronic rejection은 지속적인 면역반응으로 인하여 결국 intimal smooth muscle cell의 증식으로 미세혈관 특히 세동맥(arteriole)이 좁아져 허혈성 손상을 유발하게 되는 과정이다. 그 결과 interstitial fibrosis가 진행되고 liver graft의 경우 vanishing bile duct syndrome이 발생하게 된다.

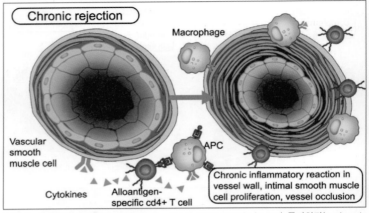

그림18. 지속적인 면역반응의 결과 vascular smooth muscle layer가 두꺼워지는 chronic rejection의 mechanism

3. Anti-rejection treatment

1) T-cell mediated rejection target 〈그림19〉

(1) T-lymphocyte depletion : anti-thymocyte globulin

(2) IL-2 receptor blocker : Basiliximab

(3) IL-2 production blocker : calcineurin inhibitor

(4) IL-2 signal blocker : mTOR inhibitor

(5) Anti-metabolite : DNA synthesis blocker

(6) Co-stimulatory signal blocker : CTLA4 Ig (Belatacept)

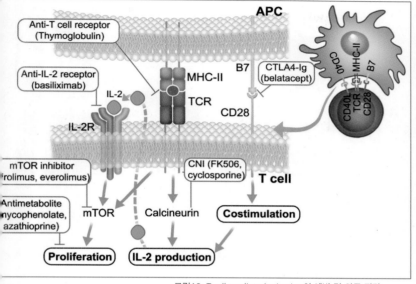

그림19. T-cell mediated rejection의 예방 및 치료 전략

2) Antibody mediated rejection target 〈그림20〉

(1) Reduce the number of cells with potential for forming more Ab
: Rituximab

(2) Physical removal of Ab : plasmapheresis

(3) Impair function of remaining Ab : IVIG (immunoglo- bulin)

(4) Reduce the number of cells with ability of Ab producing :
Bortezomib

(5) Block the complement activation through the Ab : Eculizumab

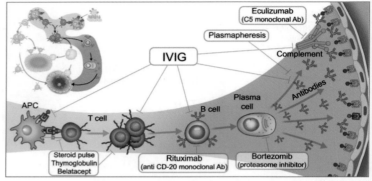

그림20. antibody mediated rejection의 예방 및 치료 전략

3) Steroid pulse therapy

   (1) Anti-inflammatory genes 활성화

   (2) Inflammatory genes 억제

   (3) mRNA stability 감소

Ⅳ. Patients evaluation and preparation

1. Cross matching test

이식을 하기 전 recipient가 donor에 대하여 얼마나 인식하고 있는지 확인하는 것은 hyperacute rejection을 예방하는 매우 중요한 과정이다. 이러한 과정은 결국 donor를 인식하는 recipient의 antibody 즉, DSA가 얼마나 존재하는가를 확인하는 과정이라고 할 수 있다. DSA의 존재를 확인하기 위한 방법은 〈그림21〉에서 보듯 여러가지가 있는데, 최근 정말로 공격성을 가지고 있는 DSA를 선별하기 위하여 보체(C1q, C3d) 와 결합한 DSA를 측정하는 방법도 제시되고 있다.

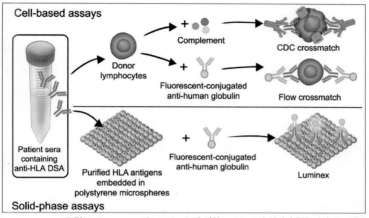

그림21. Donor specific antibody에 의한 recipient의 면역반응을 검사하는 방법

1) Complement dependent cytotoxicity (CDC)

DSA에 의하여 complement가 활성화되고 donor cell을 lysis 시키는 농도를 제시한다. 가장 강력한 anti-donor immune response의 증거이다.

2) Flow cytometry (FXM)

Donor cell에 붙은 DSA에 binding하는 형광 Ab가 형광을 발산하는 강도를 나타낸다. 역시나 강한 anti-donor response의 증거이다. 일반적으로 cross matching 양성이라는 표현은 CDC법 또는 FXM법에서 양성이 나왔을 때를 이야기한다.

3) Panel reactive antibody (PRA)

Panel에 일반적인 HLA Ag들을 깔아두고 recipient의 serum을 반응시켜 binding하는 Ab가 있는지 형광 Ab를 이용하여 확인하는 검사이다. Cross matching test에서는 양성이 나오지 않는 정도의 DSA가 존재하는 것을 확인할 수 있다.

4) Complement binding donor specific antibody (DSA)

DSA중에서도 donor cell을 공격하는 능력이 있는 DSA를 선별하기 위한 방법으로 DSA와 complement system의 일부를 같이 검사하는 방법이 제시되고 있다. 그 대상으로는 C1q, C3d, 또는 C4d가 제시되고 있다.

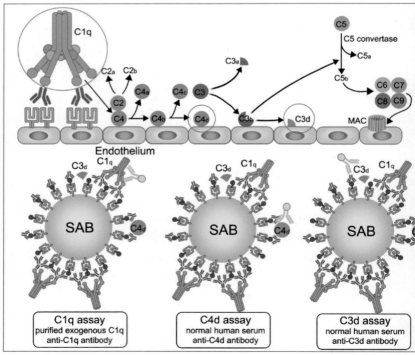

그림22. 공격성을 가지는 DSA를 선별하기 위하여 Complement binding DSA를 측정하는 방법

2. Desensitization for sensitized patients

DSA가 많거나 혈액형 부적합으로 혈액형에 대한 Ab가 존재하는 경우는 이러한 Ab를 줄여야 hyperacute rejection을 예방하고 장기적인 graft survival을 도모할 수 있다. 기본적인 방식은 antibody mediated rejection의 치료와 동일하다고 생각하면 된다.

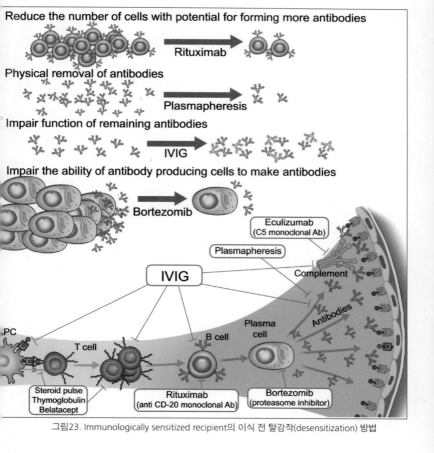

그림23. Immunologically sensitized recipient의 이식 전 탈감작(desensitization) 방법

CHAPTER 02.

IMMUNE SUPPRESSION PROTOCOL

Ⅰ. Necessity of induction therapy: prevention of acute rejection

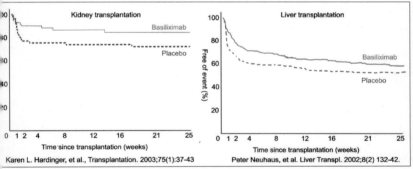

Karen L. Hardinger, et al., Transplantation. 2003;75(1):37-43

Peter Neuhaus, et al. Liver Transpl. 2002;8(2) 132-42.

☞ Comparing biopsy confirmed acute rejection events between basiliximab and placebo. Basiliximab immunoprophylaxis shows a trend toward reduction in number of acute rejection episodes in kidney and liver transplantation.

Ⅱ. The types and use of induction immunosuppressive drugs.

The types of induction immunosuppressive drugs

    (1) IL-2 receptor antibodies

       : Basiliximab, anti CD25, Simulect®

    (2) Anti lymphocyte antibodies

       : Anti thymocyte globulin (ATG) -

        Thymoglobulin (rabbit ATG®)

    (3) Anti B cell antibody:

       : anti CD20, Rituxan®, Mabthera®

1. Basiliximab (anti IL-2, anti CD25)

    1) Ix.: Routine induction in LT, Immunologic low risk patients in LDKT, SCD in DDKT

    2) Dose: 10 mg (weight <35 kg), 20 mg (weight≥35 kg)

    3) Adverse effects

       (1) GI trouble (abdominal pain, N/V, diarrhea etc.) (>10%)

       (2) Hypotension, arrhythmia (3-10%)

       (3) Leukopenia, thrombocytopenia (3-10%)

       (4) Pulmonary edema (3-10%)

    4) SMC protocol

       (1) POD #0 (after reperfusion) and POD #4 (2 times, 20 mg/time)

       (2) 대부분의 소아 LT에서는 사용하지 않으나 소아 KT에서는 사용

       (3) 학동기 recipient의 경우에는 사용하는 경우가 있기 때문에 confirm 필요

2. Rabbit anti-thymocyte globulin (rATG)

1) Ix: Immunologic intermediate and high risk group in LDKT, ECD in DDKT, Induction regimen in SPK, Refractory AR, ABOi in KT

2) Dose: 1.5 mg/kg x 3-5 days (induction: 3 days, Refractoy acute rejection: 3-5 days)

   - Decrease dose by one-half (WBC 2,000-3000 or platelet count 50,000-75,000 cells/mm^3)
   - Discontiue when WBC or platetlet count below the lower limits

3) Adverse effects

   (1) Tachycardia (23%), peripheral edema (20%), hypotension (10-16%)
   (2) Leukopenia (49-57%), thrombocytopenia (29-37%), Malignant neoplasm (4%)
   (3) Rash (8-13%), pruritis (6%)
   (4) CMV infection (13%), HSV infection (5%), sepsis (12%)
   (5) Pulmonary disease (12%), Serum sickness (7.5%)

4) rATG protocol

   (1) Before administration, body weight reduction to preop status to prevent (PRN. CRRT or HD) over 1 or 2days
   (2) Daily body weight check. If 3 kg↑, CRRT or HD apply
   (3) Daily chest AP (portable) check to prevent pulmonary edema (especially Day 1,2,3)
   (4) Daily check up for peripheral edema, neck vein distension
   (5) Daily check of ABGA at day 1-3.

5) SMC rATG 투약 schedule

(1) rATG 1.5 mg/kg with 5dw 250 mL mix via c-line over 12hrs

(2) Premedication

   ① Acetaminophen (325 mg)

- Day 1: Acetaminophen, oral administration at 30 minutes before rATG
- Day 2, 3: oral dose 325 mg q 4hr
- Day 4 ~: apply according to patient's condition (ex. BT>37.5℃, 325 mg q 4hr)

   ② Chlorpheniramine

- Day 1, 2, 3: 4 mg via iv, at 30 minutes before rATG
- Day 4 later: apply according to patient's condition

(3) Prophylaxis for opportunistic infection

   ① PJP prophylaxis 동시에 시작

- TMP-SMX 1T qd (6 months)

   ② Antifungal prophylaxis

- Itraconazole 100 mg bid (Capsule: 식사 직후 투약) 2주간 투여

   ③ Ganciclovir schedule을 동시에 시작(2주간 투여)

Ganciclovir(DHPG)				
CCr (mL/min)	Dose (mg/kg)	Dosing Interval (hrs)	유지용량 (mg/kg)	투여간격 (hrs)
>70	5	12	5.0	24
50-69	2.5	12	2.5	24
25-49	2.5	24	1.25	24
10-24	1.25	24	0.625	24
<10	1.25	투석 후 주3회	0.625	투석 후 주3회

- granulocyte $< 1,000/mm^3$ or platelet $< 20,000/mm^3$: discontinue ganciclovir

3. Rituximab (Anti B cell, anti CD20)

1) Ix.: desensitization for ABO incompatible LT and KT, Immunologic intermediate and high risk group in KT

2) Dose: 375 mg/m^2 or 200 mg

3) Adverse effects

   (1) Infection (19-62%)

   (2) Bowel obstruction/perforation (10%)

   (3) Significant cardiovascular event (arrhythmia, MI, Cardiogenic shock) (2%)

   (4) Pancytopenia (3%)

   (5) HBV reactivation (2%)

   (6) Infusion-related reaction

   ① Occurrence within 30-120 min

   ② Sx.: hypotension, angioedema, bronchospasm, urticaria

4) SMC protocol

   (1) ABO incompatible LT

   ① Dose: 375 mg/m^2 (POD# -14)

   (2) ABO incompatible KT

   ① Initianl titer≥1:256: 375 mg/m^2 (POD# -30)

   ② Initianl titer≤1:128: 200 mg (POD# -30)

   (3) According to immunologic risk in KT

   ① High risk: 375 mg/m^2 (POD# -30)

   ② Intermediate risk: 375 mg/m^2 (POD# -2)

   (4) Premedication

   ① Oral acetaminophen 650 mg

   ② IV chlorpheniramine 4 mg

(5) HLA cross-matching in LT and KT: Rituximab 투여 전과 수술 직
전 CDC, Flow cytometry 2회 시행한다

Ⅲ. The types and use of maintenance immunosuppressive drugs.

The types of maintenance immunosuppressive drugs

(1) Calcineurin inhibitors (CNI): Tacrolimus and Cyclosporine

(2) mTOR inhibitors

   ① Sirolimus (Rapamune®)

   ② Everolimus (Certican®)

(3) Anti-proliferative agents:

   ① Mycophenolate mofetil (Cellcept®, Myrept®)

   ② Mycophenolate sodium (Myfortic®)

   ③ Azathioprine

(4) Steroids

1. Tacrolimus (FK506)

약품 종류

Injection :

Prograf inj® (5 mg/1 mL/amp)

Oral agent :

Prograf®(0.5 mg, 1 mg)

Tacrobell® (0.25 mg, 0.5 mg, 1 mg)

Advagraf®(Prograf의 extended release form, 0.5 mg, 1 mg, 5 mg)

1) Ix.: First line of CNI in LT and KT recipients

2) Dose

    : 0.1-0.15 mg/kg/day in adult LT recipients

    : 0.1 mg/kg/day in KT recipients who receive MMF + Basiliximab

3) Dose adjustment: 아침 투약(7AM)직전 whole blood 내의 trough level을 측정하여 다음의 혈중 농도를 유지하도록 용량조절 특히 신기능 저하 환자(HRS, CRRT)는 투여 시기와 용량에 주의한다.

4) Adverse effects

    (1) Nephrotoxicity (less common than cyclosporine)

    (2) Neurotoxicity: mild tremor (35-55%), visual abnormalities, seizure

    (3) Hypertension

    (4) Metabolic abnormalties: DM, hyperlipidemia, hyperuricemia, hyperkalemia

    (5) GI trouble (72%)

    (6) Alopecia

5) SMC protocol

    (1) LT

        ① Start from the evening of POD #3 in usual LT recipient

        ② In patients with MELD≥25, severe infectious disease, old age, poor general condition → consider starting at POD #5 evening 1 mg

    (2) KT: start from the evening of Op day

    (3) Start 0.075 mg/kg po bid from the morning of POD #1 in pediatric recipients

6) Target Trough Level of Tacrolimus

(1) Adult LT and KT

OP~2 wk	Around 10 ng/mL
2 wk~1mon	8-10 ng/mL
After 1 month	5-8 ng/mL

(2) Pediatric LT

OP~1mon	10-12 ng/mL
1mon~3mon	8-10 ng/mL
After 3mon	5-8 ng/mL

2. Cyclosporine

약품 종류

Injection:

Cipol inj.®(250 mg/5 mL), Sandimmune inj.®(250 mg/5 mL)

Oral agent(micro-emulsion제제-소장에서의 흡수력 높임):

Cipol-N cap.®(25 mg, 100 mg), Neoral®(25 mg, 100 mg)

1) Ix.: LT and KT patients who do not tolerate tacrolimus

2) Dose: 4-10 mg/kg/day

3) Dose adjustment: 아침 투약(7AM)직전 whole blood 내의 trough level 을 측정하여 다음의 혈중 농도를 유지하도록 용량조절

4) Adverse effect

(1) Nephrotoxicity

(2) Neurotoxicity (less common than tacrolimus)

(3) Metabolic abnormalties: DM, hyperlipidemia, hyperuricemia, hyperkalemia

(4) Hepatotoxicity

(5) GI trouble (47%)

(6) Hirsutism

(7) Gingival hyperplasia

5) SMC protocol

(1) LT

① Start from the evening of POD #3 in usual LT recipient

② In patients with MELD≥25, severe infectious disease, old age, poor general condition → consider starting at POD #5 evening 1 mg

(2) KT: start from the evening of Op day

6) Target Trough Level of Cyclosporin

(1) Adult LT and KT

OP~2wk	200-250 ng/mL
1wk~3mon	150-200 ng/mL
After 3mon	Around 150 ng/mL

3. Sirolimus (Rapamune®, 0.5 mg, 1 mg, 2 mg)

1) Ix.: BK Nephritis patients after KT, CNI toxicity, De novo malignancy

• 투여 시점: BK Nephritis, serum BK DNA viral load≥4 log copies/mL

2) Dose

(1) ≥40 kg: Loading dose 6 mg on day 1; maintenance dosing 2 mg once daily

(2) <40 kg: Lodading dose 3 mg/m² on day 1; maintance dosing

$1mg/m^2$ once daily

3) Adverse effects

(1) Hyperlipidemia

(2) Proteinuria

(3) Wound dehiscence, delayed wound healing, incisional hernia

(4) Hepatic artery thrombosis after LT (most cases of HAT occurred within POD #30)

(5) Lymphocele/fluid accumulation

(6) Mouth ulcers

4) SMC protocol

(1) Loading dose: 2-6 mg a day

(2) Maintanance dose: 1-2 mg a day or 1 mg every other day

(3) Tacrolimus conversion to Sirolimus: CNI level 낮아지지 않도록 초기 투여 2~3일간 Tacrolimus와 겹쳐서 투여

(4) mTOR should not be used earlier than 30 days after LT because of HAT risk

(5) 단, 임상적판단(Sirolimus농도 등)에 따라 증, 감량할 수 있음. 또한, 초기부하용량 투여 없이 유지용량만 투여할 수 있음

4. Everolimus (Certican®, 0.25/0.5/0.75/1 mg)

1) Ix.: Renal dysfunction patients after LT, Prevention or treatment of HCC recurrence after LT

2) Dose: initially 1 mg twice daily in LT and 0.75 mg twice daily in KT

(1) If trough is < 3 ng/mL: double total daily dose

(2) If trough is > 8 ng/mL on 2 consecutive measures: decrease

dose by 0.25 mg twice daily

3) Adverse effects

(1) Metabolic effects: hyperglycemia, hyperlipidemia

(2) Generalized edema, angioedema

(3) Bone marrow suppression

(4) Hepatic artery thrombosis after LT (most cases of HAT occurred within POD #30)

(5) Graft thrombosis: an increased risk of renal artery and venous thrombosis

(6) Wound healing complication

4) SMC protocol

	간기능 정상	경증 간기능 장애 (Child-Pugh A)	중등도 간기능 장애 (Child-Pugh B)	중증 간기능 장애 (Child-Pugh C)
LT	1일 2회 1 mg	1일 2회 0.75 mg	1일 2회 0.5 mg	1일 2회 0.25 mg

5) Tacrolimus, Everolimus 동시 요법에서만 국내승인

5. Mycophenolate mofetil : Cellcept® (250 mg), Myrept cap® (250 mg/500 mg)
Mycophenolate sodium : Myfortic® (180 mg/360 mg)

1) Ix.: LT and KT recipients

2) Dose: 750 mg twice a day (MMF), 540 mg twice a day (Mycophenolate sodium)

3) Adverse effect

(1) Leukopenia (19-46%), anemia (20-45%), thromobocyto-penia (24-38%)

(2) Severe neutropenia (2-4%)

      (3) GI trouble (20-50%): abdominal pain, N/V, ileus, diarrhea

      (4) Carviovascular: HTN (18-79%), edema (17-68%), hypotension (34%)

  4) SMC protocol (starting dose and dose reduction)

      (1) POD #1 morning, 750 mg (540 mg) twice a day in LT

      (2) POD #3 morning, 500 mg (360 mg) twice a day in MELD≥25 LT

      (3) OP day evening, 750 mg (540 mg) twice a day in KT

      (4) 300 mg/m^2 (BSA) po bid in pediatric recipient (드물게 사용)

      (5) Leukopenia → dose reduction 고려

      (6) Active infection (CMV, HZV, sepsis, pneumonia 등) or severe adverse effect → dose reduction or D/C

  5) Myfortic : Patients with severe GI trouble, instead of MMF
Mycophenolic acid (MPA) level monitoring : no routine f/u in LT, weekly f/u in KT, Target trough level: 1~3 ng/mL

  6) Mycophenolate mofetil 250 mg (1 cap) = Mycophenolate sodium 180 mg (1 tab)

6. Azathioprine (Immuran®)

  1) Ix.: Pregnant patients → lower doses (<2 mg/kg/day) are recommended)

  2) Dose

      (1) If used with steroids alone, a suitable dose is 2.5 mg/kg/day

      (2) 1.5 mg/kg, or 100 mg/day is standard dose in triple-therapy

  3) Adverse effect

      (1) Bone marrow suppression: leukopenia (>50%), throm-

bocytopenia (5%)

(2) GI trouble (23%): anorexia, N/V, diarrhea

(3) Pancreatitis

(4) Hepatotoxicity

(5) Hair loss

(6) Squamous cell carcinoma

4) SMC protocol

(1) 3 mg/kg/day to 5 mg/kg/day single dose given at time of transplantation

(2) 1 mg/kg/day to 3 mg/kg/day for maintenance

(3) dose usually adjusted depending on WBCs

(4) lower doses should be considered in presence of renal dysfunction

7. Steroid

1) Ix.: LT and KT recipients

2) Dose: Steroid use varies among transplant centers

3) Adverse effect

(1) Skin thinning and ecchymosis, cushingoid feature, acne, weight gain

(2) Ophthalmologic effects: cataracts, increased intraocular pressure, exophthalmos

(3) Cardiovascular effects: fluid retention, HTN, premature atherosclerotic disease

(4) Bone effects: osteoporosis, osteonecrosis (avascular or ischemic necrosis of bone)

(5) Hyperglycemia

(6) HPA axis suppression

4) SMC protocol in Adults

POD	0	1	2	3	4	5-7	8-14	15-1m	1-3m
MPD dose (mg)	500 IV	500 IV	250 IV	125 IV	75 IV	60 IV	16 po bid	8 po bid	4 po bid
PD does (mg)							20 po bid	10 po bid	5 po bid

(1) Tapering & cessation should be decided based on individual condition of recipients (usually around POD 3 months)

(2) MELD $\geq$ 25, status I and IIA: early tapering

5) SMC protocol in Pediatric

POD	0	1	2	3	4	5	6-7	8-1mon
MPD dose (mg/kg)	20 IV	10 IV	8 IV	6 IV	4 IV	2 IV	1 IV	
PD does (mg/kg)								0.15 po bid

(1) Tapering & cessation should be decided based on individual condition of recipients (usually around POD 1 months)

6) Steroid potency/Conversion chart

Agent	Equivalent dose(mg)	Glucocorticoid potency	Mineralocorticoid potency	Half-life (hrs)
Cortisone	25	0.8	2	8-12
Hydrocortisone (Corti solu)	20	1	2	8-12
MPD	4	5	0.5	18-36
Prednisone	5	4	1	18-36
Prednisolone	5	4	1	18-36
Dexamethasone	0.75	25	0	36-54

IV. Treatment for Acute Rejection

1. Steroid (SPT, Steroid pulse therapy): as postop. Methylprednisolone

1) Schedule

(1) Adults (> 40 kg);

- Bolus (3 days) - 500 mg IV qd
- Then taper to 250, 125, 75, 60 mg IV qd
- Resume oral MPD at maintenance dose

LT/PT		
TMP-SMX	1T qd daily for 6 weeks	Protozoa, P. jiroveci
Itraconazole	100mg bid for 4 weeks	Fungus other than P. jiroveci
No ganciclovir	CMV pre-emptive CMV antigenemia monitor for 12 weeks	CMV

KT		
TMP-SMX	1T qd daily for 6 weeks	Protozoa, P. jiroveci
No Itraconazole	None	Fungus other than P. jiroveci
No ganciclovir	CMV pre-emptive CMV antigenemia monitor for 12 weeks	CMV

(2) Children (< 40 kg);

- Bolus (3days) 10-20 mg/kg IV, and then tapering (daily half dose)
- Resume oral PD at maintenance (0.15 mg/kg po bid)
- Ganciclovir start (CMV prophylaxis): resume PO acyclovir with po PD

- Anti-ulcer medication (Intravenous H2 blocker)
- CNI level: 점차 올려 SPT 끝날 때 10 ng/mL로 유지
- CMV antigenemia check 월,수,금

(3) 예) 500-500-500-250-125-75-60 mg (Methylprednisolone IV)으로 감량한 후 8일째부터 MPD 16 mg bid 3일간, 8 mg bid 3일로 tapering 하면서 가장 최근 dose에 도달하도록 한다.

(4) Mini SPT

500-250-125-75-60 이후 동일.

2) 주의사항

(1) 보통 biopsy 결과 확인 후에 SPT를 시행하나, 임상적으로 rejection 이 의심될 때 일찍 시작하는 것도 고려한다.

(2) Biopsy 하는 경우 autoimmune lab과 ABO-I이면 PRA screening 을 같이 처방.

(3) KT 환자에서 수술 후 2주 이내 rejection이 생긴 경우 HLA Ab Single Identification, PRA (Class I/II)를 시행한다.

(4) KT 환자에서 AMR (Antibody mediated rejection)을 시사할 경우 IVIG 추가 투여를 고려한다.

(5) SPT 시작과 동시에 TMP-SMX 1T qd daily 시작. 이후 5주 유지 after SPT(총 6주)

(6) LT 환자에서 HCV, HBV recur 환자는 정확한 biopsy 확인이 필요하다. Hepatitis C는 조직검사를 하더라도 rejection과 구별이 힘들고 SPT는 치명적 결과를 가져올 수 있다.

(7) SPT시 - ulcer medication (Intravenous H2 blocker)와 Chest X-ray, BST 반드시 check 한다.

(8) CNI trough level : cyclosporine around 200 ng/mL , tacrolimus around 10 ng/mL ⇨ 유지바람

2. Second Rescue: Steroid-unresponsive group- rATG

: "면역억제제의 종류와 용법" 참조

(1) Rejection치료기간 동안 기존의 Steroid는 주지 않음 (SPT와 동일 한 schedule로 투여함)

(2) Tacrolimus, cyclosporin, MMF는 환자 상태에 따라 중단하거나 low dose로 사용.

(3) Antifungal prophylaxis: Itraconazole 사용

3. Intra Venous Immune Globulin (IVIG) Therapy

(1) Ix.

① AMR : Bx.에서 AMR 소견/C4d positive/DSA (+) 중 2가지 이상

② highly sensitized patient의 induction 시에 투여 고려

③ Severe anemia with parvovirus infection in kidney recipients

(2) Premedication: Chloropheniramine 4 mg ivs

(3) Start with 0.01~0.02 mL/kg/min for 30 min (0.6~1.2 mL/kg/hr)

→ Increase up to 0.02~0.04 mL/kg/min (1.2~2.4 mL/kg/hr)

Ex〉 50kg 환자의 경우 30 mg/hr로 30분간 투여 시작. 이후 부작용 없다면 30분마다 60→90→120 mg/hr 까지 증량하여 투여하며 부작용 발생 시 1단계 낮춰서 투여

(4) Side effect: shock, flushing, fever, dizziness, nausea, headache, hypotension, elevated AST/ALT, BUN/Cr

① Close observation: Vital sign

② Prepare epinephrine injection for anaphylaxis

③ Prn) use of analgesics for headache

CHAPTER 03.

INFECTION IN TRANSPLANT RECIPIENTS

I. Pre-Transplant evaluation for infectious disease

1. Recipient evaluation and management

1) History taking: 최근 1년 이내 감염증으로 치료받은 이력, 과거 결핵 치료력 등

2) Radiologic test: chest PA/PNS series, abnormal finding이 있을 경우 chest CT/OMU CT고려

3) Serologic assay: HBsAg, anti-HBs Ab, anti-HBc Ab (IgG), HBeAg, anti-HBe Ab, anti-HCV Ab (IgG), anti-HAV (IgG), RPR, anti-HIV combo, CMV Ab (IgG), EB-VCA (IgG), VZV Ab (IgG), HSV Type 1 & 2 Ab (IgG), Toxoplasma Ab (IgG), Measles Ab (IgG)

4) KT recipeint: Polyomavirus type BK DNA PCR, Parvovirus B19 DNA PCR (이식 전일)

5) PCR: HBV DNA Quantitation (HBV+환자), HBV YMDD mutation (HBV antivral medication중인 경우), HCV RNA detection (HCV+환자), HCV genotype (HCV+환자)

6) Cultures: Blood Culture 3 pairs, Gram stain & culture (Urine, Throat, Sputum, Stool), Fungus culture (Urine, Throat, Sputum, Stool)

7) MDR pathogen screening: Nasal MRSA culture, VRE rectal screening, CRE screening (rectal swab), Carbapenemase gene PCR (rectal swab)

8) Parasite: Stool exam

9) Latent TB w/u
   (1) TB Specific Interferon-Gamma (QFT) 시행, TB Hx 에 대해 history taking
   (2) QFT positive, TB Hx, or old TB lesion on CXR: non-contrast Chest CT check
   (3) QFT inderminate: TB Specific Interferon-Gamma (T-SPOT) 추가 검사
   (4) 상기 검사나 Hx상 positive finding이 있는경우 LTBI 치료 필요성에 대해 감염내과 협진

10) Vaccination
   (1) 과거 vaccination Hx확인: Pneumococcal, Tdap, Zoster, Influenza
   (2) Organ failure가 진행하면 immunogencity가 감소하므로 가능한 환자가 stable할 때 일찍 접종
   (3) 이식 전 vaccination은 사백신의 경우 이식 2주 전, 생백신 (Varicella, Zoster, MMR)의 경우 이식 4주 전까지 완료

(4) 동일 부위 접종 시 local reaction 확인을 위해 3 cm 이상 간격을 둠

(5) 이식 전 vaccination이 시행되지 못한 경우 및 추가 접종은 이식 3 개월 후 clinically stable할 때 시행. 단, influenza vaccination은 유행시기를 놓칠 수 있으므로 이식 1개월 후부터 접종 가능.

(6) Universal vaccine

: Influenza (IM) - October to April

Pneumococcal: PCV13 (IM) and PPSV23 (IM)

- PCV13을 먼저 접종하고, 8주 뒤 PPSV23을 접종
- PPV23의 경우 5년 뒤 추가 접종이 필요

Tdap (Tetanus, Diphtheria, Acelluar, Pertussis, IM)

- 50세 (1958년 이전 출생자) 이상에서는 Td (XTD, IM) 2차 (1개 월 뒤), 3차 (6개월 뒤) 고려

Zoster vaccine (SC)

- 50세 이상 환자에서 이식일로부터 4주 이상 여유가 있는 경우 고려
- 현재 국내에서 사용 가능한 Zoster vaccine (Zostavax®)은 생백신으로, 이식일까지 충분한 여유가 있을 때 접종하는 것 이 바람직하며 HCC로 인해 LDLT를 대기하거나 DDLT가능성 이 있는 LC 환자들의 경우 이식일이 예정일보다 당겨질 수 있 으므로 접종에 주의가 필요함. Recombiant zoster vaccine 인 Shingrix®는 사백신으로, 미국 FDA approval을 획득하고 solid organ transplant (SOT) recipient 를 대상으로 study 진 행 중인 상태로 아직 국내에 출시되지 않았으나 추후 도입 가 능성이 높음.

(7) Special considerations

  : HAV A IgG negative

- Hepatitis A vaccine (IM) 1회 접종, 6~12개월 뒤 2차 접종

  HBsAb negative

- Hepatitis B vaccine (IM) 1회 접종, 1달 뒤 HBsAb f/u하여 항체 Boosting 유무를 확인하고 음성일 경우 2차 (1달 뒤), 3차 (6개월 뒤) 접종 시행 1달 뒤 HBsAb을 f/u

  VZV Ab (IgG) negative

- 이식일로부터 4주 이상 여유가 있는 경우 Varicella vaccine (SC) 1회 접종 필요

  Measles Ab (IgG) negative

- 이식일로부터 4주 이상 여유가 있는 경우 MMR vaccine (SC) 1회 접종 필요

11) 다양한 경우의 수가 있을 수 있으므로 감염내과 협진하여 vaccination 진행하고, emergency OP로 pre-evaluation 또는 vaccination이 시행되지 못한 경우에는 이식 후 퇴원 전 감염협진을 보거나 퇴원 후 post OP 3개월 시점에 감염내과 외래 f/u

II. Post-Transplant management of infection

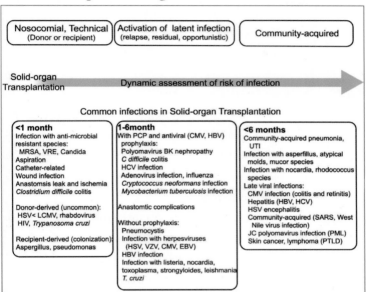

Fishman JA. N Engl J Med 2007;357:2601-14

1. Postoperative Routine Surveillance

1) Ordinary Bacteria and Fungus

(1) Blood culture, Gram stain and culture (urine, sputum, drains, bile, wounds), Fungus culture (urine, sputum, drains, bile, wounds)

- Routine post OP f/u - POD #1, #3, #5
- 발열이나 CRP 상승, unstable V/S, drainage fluid의 color change 등 infection이 의심될 경우 이전 검사일에 상관없이 f/u

- 임상적으로 안정된 상태에서 drainage 유지할 경우 주 1~2회 drainage fluid에 대한 culture f/u

(2) Infection이 의심될 경우 경험적 항생제의 시작 또는 변경 고려

(3) 항생제 선택에 대해서 필요 시 감염내과 협진

2) CMV

   (1) CMV antigenemia surveillance

- Immediate Post-Op recipient, high-risk recipients, antigenemia positive recipients or CMV disease recipients

  : frequently f/u (on Mon., Wed., Fri. - for a week after transplantation)

- Weekly while hospitalized

- After discharge, at every visit (q 4 weeks) till post-op. 12 weeks

- In case of fever or leukopenia of unknown cause

- Follow-up examination without CMV infection

  a. Every Mon., Wed., Fri. until discharge

  b. Once a week if readmission after transplantation (in hospital stay)

  c. Once a month until 12 weeks after transplantation (when OPD f/u)

Every Mon., Wed., Fri. if ganciclovir on medication because of CMV infection (on preemptive treatment) or on Steroid pulse therapy

3) EBV

   (1) EBV-VCA (IgG/IgM), EBV-EA, EBNA

  : less reliable for post-transplant surveillance

(2) EBV Quantitative PCR

- High-risk patients
    a. Transplant from EBV IgG (+) donor to EBV IgG (-) recipient
    b. All children < 1 yr regardless of pretransplant serology
- PreOp ~ PostOp 1 yr - every 1 month
    ~ PostOp 2 yr - q 2 months
    이후 - q 4 months

4) HBV: Hepatitis profile, HBV DNA Quantitation

5) HCV: HCV RNA Detection, HCV RNA Quantitation

2. Prevention and treatment of infection

Overview of prophylactic antimicrobial

Antimicrobial	Dosage and duration	Target
LT		
Cefotaxime	2.0 g IV q 8hrs ×2 days	Bacterial
Ampicillin/ Sulbactam	3.0 g IV q 6hrs ×2 days	
TMP-SMX	1T qd, POD#5 to 6 months	Protozoa P. jiroveci
Itraconazole	Syrup: 100 mg bid during NPO (tube feeding시 공복에 투약) Capsule: 100 mg bid (with meal) until POD#30	Fungus other than P. jiroveci
Gangiclovir in high risk * D IgG(+)/R IgG(-)	IV ganciclovir 5 mg/kg iv q24h →Valganciclovir po 900 mg qd until POD#100	CMV

HBIG in HBsAg (+)	10,000 U, OPday-POD#6 (7 times) Weekly until 4th week (3 times) Monthly until 12 month Injection based on HBsAb titer, thereafter * in HBV-DNA (+) or HBeAg (+) recipient 20,000 U, OPday~POD#6 (7 times), the rest is same	HBV
HBIG in donor HBcAb (+)	10,000 U, OPday~POD#6 (7 times). Injection based on HBsAb titer, thereafter	
Antiviral for HBV	Keep the med if the recipient was under antiviral Entecavir 0.5 mg qd, (POD#1~), when no previous meds or cessation after serocoversion	

KT

Cefotaxime	2.0 g IV q 8hrs ×2 days	Bacterial
TMP-SMX	1T qd, POD#5 to 6 months	Protozoa P. jiroveci
Itraconazole in ATG induction	Syrup: 100 mg bid during NPO (tube feeding시 공복에 투약) Capsule: 100 mg bid (2W) until POD#14	Fungus other than P. jiroveci
Ganciclovir in high risk * D IgG (+)/R IgG (-)	IV ganciclovir 5 mg/kg iv q24h →Valganciclovir po 900 mg qd until POD#200	CMV
Ganciclovir in ATG induction	IV ganciclovir 5 mg/kg iv q24h For 2 weeks	

PT/SPKT

Cefotaxime	2.0 g IV q 8hrs ×2 days	Bacterial
Ampicillin/ Sulbactam	3.0 g IV q 6hrs ×2 days	
TMP-SMX	1T qd, POD#5 to 6 months	Protozoa P. jiroveci
itraconazole in ATG induction	Syrup: 100 mg bid during NPO (tube feeding시 공복에 투약) Capsule: 100 mg bid (with meal) until POD#14	Fungus other than P. jiroveci

Gangiclovir in high risk * D IgG (+)/R IgG (-)	IV ganciclovir 5 mg/kg iv q24h →Valganciclovir po 900 mg qd until POD#200 (SPKT) POD#100 (PT)	CMV
Ganciclovir in ATG induction	IV ganciclovir 5 mg/kg iv q24h For 2 weeks	

1) Bacterial and protozoal infections

   (1) Prophylaxis

   ① Bacterial prophylaxis

   i) Systemic antibiotics

   (i) LT

   : Cefotaxime 2.0 g IV q 8hr (AST) (pediatric 30-40 mg/kg) and Ampicillin/Sulbactam 3 g IV q 6hr (AST) (pediatric 50 mg/kg)

   (ii) KT

   : Cefotaxime 2 g iv q 8hr

   (iii) Start with induction

   (iv) Reinjection intraoperatively in case of prolonged surgery

   (v) Duration: until POD#2 in LT and KT recipients

   (vi) If the recipient has antibiotics before surgery with sepsis, keep it. Consult with infection department.

   ii) Prophylactic antibiotics during procedures

   (i) Cefotaxime and Ampicillin/sulbactam with invasive procedures (for 2~3 days)

   (ii) Cholangiography, ERBD, ENBD, angiography, balloon

dilatation, stent insertion, biopsy, etc.

(iii) 최근 3개월 이내 biliary tract이나 blood에서 resistant pathogen이 동정된 이력이 있는 경우에는 그에 맞추어 예방적 항생제를 선택 (필요 시 감염내과 협진).

(iv) Cholangitis/Abscess가 의심되지 않는 환자에서 PTBD/PCD insertion시 예방적 항생제는 적응증이 되지 않으나, infection이 의심되는 경우에는 예상되는 pathogen에 대한 targeted therapy를 시행 (이전 동정력 고려).

② Toxoplasma prophylaxis

i) Toxoplasma IgG D+/R- or R+

ii) TMP-SMX 1T p.o qd until 6mo. after transplantation.

(2) Bacterial infection

① Vancomycin-resistant enterococcus (Nellore et al., Clin Transplant, 2019,33(9),e13549)

i) Transplant clinicians should have a high index of suspicion for VRE infection, particularly in VRE-colonized patients and SOT recipients with suspected or confirmed intra-abdominal infections (strong, low).

ii) Ampicillin is the treatment of choice for ampicillin-susceptible VRE infections (strong, low).

iii) Linezolid and daptomycin (8-10 mg/kg) are both first-line treatment choices for ampicillin-resistant VRE bloodstream and other invasive infections (strong, moderate).

iv) Treatment should be discontinued when clinical stability and source control have been achieved (strong, low).

v) Arbitrary prolonged treatment durations (eg, "2-6 weeks") should be avoided except for infective endocarditis. Infective endocarditis resulting from VRE should be treated for at least 6 weeks (strong, low).

vi) The need for VRE contact precautions, particularly in an outbreak setting, should be determined in collaboration with the hospital epidemiologist (strong, moderate)

vii) Comment〉〉 SMC protocol에서는 Donor/recipient에서 VRE screening을 시행하고 있으며 VRE carrier에 대해서 Cohort 격리 및 contact precaution을 시행하고 있음. VRE carriage rate는 철저한 접촉주의 및 손위생으로 control이 가능함. VRE 는 virulence가 낮아 immunocompetent host에서는 clinical infection을 잘 일으키지 않으나, 1) 수술 시 biliary tree의 breakage가 일어나며, 2) JP나 PTBD 등의 foreign body를 유치하는 경우가 많으며, 3) 면역억제제를 사용하는 LT환자에서는 VRE infection이 쉽게 일어나며 장기간 항생제 치료가 필요한 경우가 많음. 국내 VRE strain의 대부분은 Enterococcus faecium이며 multi-drug resistance를 보여 Ampicillin이 실제 사용가능 한 경우는 드묾. Enterococcus gallinarum의 경우 Van C gene을 encode하여 Vancomycin reistance를 보이며, 이 경우 Ampicillin이 susceptible한 경우 Ampicillin으로 치료가 가능함. 현재 국내 Daptomycin이 도입되어 있지 않아 VRE bacteremia가 발생하였을 경우의 TOC 는 Linezolid임. Linezolid는 Blood, CSF등 sterile fluid 에서 VRE가 동정되는 경우에만 보험 적용이 가능함. 복강내 감염의 경우 Tigecylcine 이 현재 TOC이나, Tigecycline은 혈중농도가 낮아 인해 Bacteremia가 있는 경우 1차로 추천되지 않음.

② Multidrug-resistant Gram negative bacteria (Treatment recommendation in supplement)

(Pouch et al., Clin Transplant, 2019,33(9),e13594)

  i) ESBL-producing Enterobacteriaceae (ESBL-EB)

    (i) Resistance: extended-spectrum penicillins, aztreonam, and 3rd-generation cephalosporins

    (ii) in vitro susceptibility: cephamycins (cefoxitin, cefmetazole, and cefotetan), carbapenems, and β-lactamase inhibitor (eg, clavulanic acid, sulbactam, and tazobactam).

    (iii) Treatment

      - Carbapenem, drug of choice for ESBLEB infections (strong, high).

      - 1st-gen β-lactam/β-lactamase inhibitor, including Piperacillin/Tazobactam, should not be used as 1st line (strong, high).

    (iv) Prevention

      - Contact precautions (strong, moderate).

      - Intestinal decolonization for ESBL-EB, not recommended (strong, moderate).

      - Donors with ESBL-EB should receive effective antimicrobial therapy for 24-48 hours prior to procurement. In the setting of donor bacteremia or infection of the organ being transplanted, recipients should receive at least a 7-day course of antibiotics targeting the donor ESBL-EB isolate (weak, low).

   (v) Comment>> 현재 국내에서는 ESBL producing Entero-bacteriacea에 대한 접촉 주의는 시행하지 못하고 있음. Donor가 ESBL producing Enterobacteriacea를 포함한 Drug-resistant pathogen을 carriage하는 경우에는 예방적 항생제 선택에 대해 감염내과 협진이 필요함. 최근 RCT에서 ESBL producing Enterobacteriacea bacteremia treatment outcome이 Piperacillin/Tazobactam에 비해 Carbapenem이 우월하게 보고되어 guideline에서는 Carbapenem을 TOC로 권고하고 있으나, Piperacillin/Tazobactam에 대한 감수성이 좋은 경우 중증도에 따라 Piperacillin/Tazobactam으로 치료가 가능함.

ii) Carbapenem-resistant Enterobacteriaceae (CRE)

   (i) Resistance: Carbapenemases are a heterogeneous group of enzymes conferring resistance to carbapen-ems

   (ii) Treatment

    - When susceptible, Ceftazidime/avibactam (strong, moderate) and Meropenem/vaborbactam (strong, low) monotherapy for CRE infections.

    - Therapeutic options for MBL-producing Enterobacter-iaceae include combination therapy with Ceftazidime/avibactam and aztreonam (strong, low)

    - Carbapenem-containing combination regimens have been associated with improved outcomes compared to noncarbapenem-containing regimens in the management of invasive CRE infections; however, carbapenem-containing regimens are not recommended if the meropenem MIC ≥ 4 $\mu g/mL$ (strong, moderate).

- Tigecycline, not recommended as monotherapy for CRE. Inability to achieve adequate serum or urine concentrations and the association with excess mortality (strong, low).

(iii) Prevention

- History of CRE colonization or infection is not a contradindication for transplantation based upon this factor alone (strong, moderate).

- Intestinal decolonization with known CRE carriage is not recommended (strong, moderate).

- Recipients with organs from bacteremic donors or from donors with colonization or infection of the allograft should receive at least 7 days of targeted antimicrobial therapy (strong, moderate).

(iv) Comment〉〉 SMC protocol에서는 Donor/recipient에서 CRE screening과 Carbapenemase gene PCR 검사를 시행하고 있으며, (Carbapenemase-producing Enterobacteriacaea, CPE) carrier의 경우 1인실 격리를 시행하고 있음. Carbapenemase gene을 가지지 않고 다른 기전으로 carbapenem에 내성을 보이는 경우도 접촉주의가 필요하나, Carbapenemase gene을 가지고 있는 CPE의 경우 전파력이 강하여 각별한 주의가 필요함. 2010년대에 들어 국내에서도 CPE outbreak이 발생하였고, outbreak control을 위해 ICU를 폐쇄하였던 경우도 수 차례 있었

음. CRE는 대부분 multi-drug resistance를 보여 clinical infection이 발생하였을 때 사용가능한 항생제가 제한적임. Amikacin이나 Colistin 등 nephrotoxic agent사용이 필요한 경우가 많으며, Ceftazidime/avibactam 등 Drug-resistant Enterobacteriaceae를 target으로 한 항생제가 새로 개발되고 있으나 아직 국내 사용이 제한적임.

iii) MDR, XDR, and PDR pseudomonas aeruginosa

   (i) Resistance: ESBLs, carbapenemases, particularly Metallo β-lactamase, and expanded-spectrum class D-β-lactamases, have also been identified in P aeruginosa isolates

   (ii) Treatment

   - The routine use of combination therapy for P aeruginosa remains controversial. However, in suspected infection with XDR or PDR P aeruginosa, we recommend empiric combination therapy (strong, moderate).

   - β-lactams should be administered as high-dose continuous-infusion therapy as able to optimize pharmacokinetics (strong, moderate).

   - When susceptible, Ceftolozane/tazobactam can be used in the treatment of MDR and XDR P aeruginosa infections. Ceftolozane/tazobactam should be administered at a higher dose (equivalent of 3 g intravenously every 8 hours) for pseudomonal pneumonia (strong, moderate).

- Adjunctive inhaled colistin or tobramycin is recommended for the treatment of pseudomonal pneumonia (weak, low).

(iii) Prevention

- Patients harboring MDR, XDR, and PDR P aeruginosa should be placed in contact isolation (strong, moderate).

(iv) Comment〉〉 Ceftolozane/tazobactam은 현재 국내에서 비급여로 사용가능한 상태이나, 추후 급여 기준 신설 가능성 있음.

iv) Carbapenem-resistant acinetobacter baumannii (CRAB)

(i) Treatment

- Carbapenem and polymyxin combination therapy is associated with microbiologic eradication of CRAB and can be used to treat CRAB infections (strong, moderate)

- High-dose sulbactam (≥9 g/d) can be used in the treatment of CRAB infections (weak, low)

- Inhaled colistin can be used as an adjunct to systemic therapy or as monotherapy in nonbacteremic respiratory infections (weak, moderate).

- Minocycline is an alternative, as monotherapy or combination therapy, for infections with CRAB (weak, low).

(ii) Prevention

- Contact precautions (strong, moderate).

- In the setting of an outbreak, evaluation for a potential common source should be pursued and compliance with hand hygiene, environmental disinfection, and device care should be assessed and evaluated for improvement (strong, moderate).

(iii) Comment〉〉CRAB 복강내 감염의 경우 Tigecycline이 감수성으로 보고되는 경우에는 투약 가능하며, 중증감염이나 폐렴의 경우 Colistin을 사용해야 하는 경우가 많음. Minocyclin의 경우 국내 IV formulation이 도입되어 있지 않아 중증감염에서의 사용은 제한적임.

2) Fungal infections

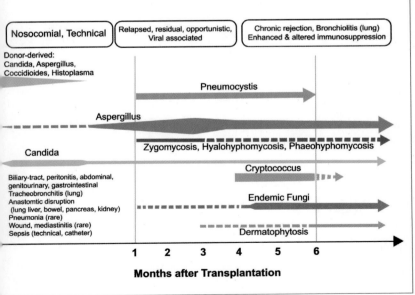

그림. Timeline of post-transplant fungal infection

(1) Prophylaxis for fungal infection

① Pneumocystis infection prophylaxis (Pneumocystis jirovecii)

  i)   Adult LT & KT

      (i)   TMP-SMX (Bactrim) 1T p.o qd until 6 mo. after transplantation.

      (ii) Start medication at POD#5.

      (iii) If the immunosuppressant is to be increased due to acute rejection even after 6 mo of transplantation, consider bactrim administration for additional 2-3 mo.

      (iv) Bactrim을 복용하지 못하는 경우에는 alternative agent (e.g pentamidine nebulizer)에 대해 감염내과 협진

  ii) Pediatric dose: 150 mg/750 mg/m^2/day

  → SMC protocol; divide two as bactrim syrup(8 mg/40 mg/cc)

② Prevention of other fungal infection

  i)   LT, KT with ATG induction (SPK 포함)

      (i)   Itraconazole syrup 100 mg bid (adult), 2.5 mg/kg bid (ped) (during NPO)- Syrup은 공복에 복용한다

      (ii) If the patient start diet, continue itraconazole 100 mg bid (till POD#30 for LT, POD#14 for KT with ATG induction/SPK). - Capsule은 식사와 함께 복용한다

      (iii) Continue the same dosage if the patient has risks of invasive aspergillosis (itraconazole 100 mg bid)

      (iv) Pediatric dosage: 2.5 mg/kg bid

            If fungal Infection is suspected during itraconazole medication, consult with the infectious disease department to select an empirical antifungal agent

(2) Candida infection

   ① Risk factors for Candida infections

     i)   "net state of immunosuppression"

     ii) Abdominal transplant recipients: due to colonization of the GI tract

         (i)   Anastomotic leakage

         (ii) Repeat laparotomy

         (iii) Choledochojejunostomy in LT

     iii) Older age

     iv) Broad-spectrum antibiotic therapy

     v)   Central venous catheter

     vi) Parenteral nutrition

     vii) Prolonged neutropenia

     viii) Prolonged ICU stay

     ix) DM

     x)   Renal replacement therapy

   ② Clinical presentations: nonspecific, range from only abnormal lab to septic shock

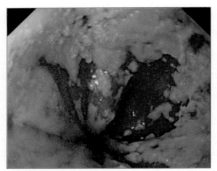

그림. Candida esophagitis

③ Diagnosis: culture or visualization of organism in tissue histopathology

● Key recommendations (Aslam et al., Clin Transplant, 33(9), e13623, 2019)

   i) Blood cultures, sterile tissue/fluid cultures, and histopathology, when appropriate, should be obtained in patients suspected of having invasive candidiasis (strong, moderate).

   ii) Use of non-culture based methods such as 1,3 beta-d glucan or T2 Candida assay is recommended in SOT recipients for the diagnosis of Invasive candidiasis if culture and/or histopathology of tissue are not available or negative (weak, low).

   iii) Antifungal susceptibility testing for azole resistance is recommended for all bloodstream and clinically relevant Candida isolates. Testing for echinocandin resistance in patients previously treated with an echinocandin and for C glabrata, C parapsilosis, and C auris isolates is also recommended (strong, low).

iv) Comment〉〉 현재 국내에 Beta-D glucan assay가 도입되었으나 specificity가 낮아 Beta-D glucan assay결과 단독으로 Candida 치료의 근거로 삼기는 어려움. SMC에서는 Blood culture에서 동정된 Candida species에 대해서는 Antifungal drug sensitivity test (DST)를 routine하게 시행하나, bile/urine 등 non-sterile specimen에서는 DST를 시행하지 않으므로, 임상적으로 의미가 있는 경우에는 Antifugnal DST를 추가로 의뢰하여야 함.

④ Treatment (see Supplement)

● Three classes of antifungal agents: Azoles (fluconazole, voriconazole, etc.): echinocandins (anidulafungin, caspofungin and micafungin): and polyenes (amphotericin B deoxycholate and lipid formulation of amphotericin B)

　i) Considerations in choosing agents during empirical therapy

　　(i) prior exposure to antifungal agents or empirical therapy within the past 90 days may portend resistance.

　　(ii) C. glabrata may manifest reduced susceptibility to fluconazole and higher doses may be necessary for effective treatment

　　(iii) C krusei is resistant to fluconazole

　　(iv) Echinocandins are less active against C parapsilosis

(v) Echinocandins achieve therapeutic concentrations in most body sites except the eye, central nervous system, and the urine although there are reports of their efficacy in candiduria and candidemia due to a Candida urinary tract infection.

- Key recommendations (Aslam et al., Clin Transplant, 33(9), e13623, 2019)

  i) Early initiation of antifungal with suspected/confirmed IC is recommended (strong, moderate)

  ii) An echinocandin is recommended for initial treatment of candidemia and invasive candidiasis (strong, high).

  iii) Fluconazole is recommended as alternative if the pathogen is likely to be fluconazole susceptible, and not critically ill (strong, high).

  iv) Echinocandin to fluconazole transition is recommended in stable patient when isolate is fluconazole susceptible, and bloodstream has cleared (strong, moderate).

  v) Echinocandin to oral voriconazole transition is recommended for fluconazole-resistant but voriconazole susceptible isolates (strong, low).

  vi) Treatment duration for candidemia: at least 2 weeks "after clearance" of the bloodstream and removal of infected central venous catheters (strong, moderate).

  vii) Treatment duration for invasive candidiasis: at least 2 weeks and potentially longer until resolution of all signs and symptoms of invasive candidiasis (strong, moderate).

viii) Central venous catheters should be removed if possible in candidemia (strong, moderate).

ix) Esophageal candidiasis: Fluconazole is recommended as initial therapy. When refractory to fluconazole, voriconazole or posaconazole are recommended as alternative (strong, high).

x) Asymptomatic candiduria: Should not be treated unless the patient is to undergo cystoscopy with stent removal where treatment for up to 7 days is recommended (strong, low).

xi) Candida isolated from the respiratory tract represents colonization and should not be treated except in lung transplant recipients with Candida tracheobronchitis (strong, moderate).

xii) Empiric antifungal for suspected IC in the setting of persistent fever, Candida colonization, and other risk factors for IC may be initiated with an echinocandin if hemodynamically unstable or fluconazole if hemodynamically stable for a duration of up to 2 weeks in the absence of an alternative diagnosis (strong, low).

xiii) Comment〉〉 현재 국내에서 Candidiasis치료시 Invasive candidiasis가 증명된 중증환자(icu care)에서만 Echinocandin이 보험 인정 됨. 중증 환자가 아닐 경우 Fluconazole과 Conventional amphotericin B이 1차 약제로 인정되나, Conventional amphotericin B는 renal toxicity등의 S/E로 인하여 사용이 제한됨. 1차 치료에 fail하거나 약제내

성이 확인이 된 경우 감염내과 협진을 통하여 voriconazole이 나 echinocandin 등의 항진균제 사용이 가능함. Voriconazole 의 경우 FK506과의 drug interaction에 주의하여야 하며 drug level monitoring이 필요함.

⑤ Therapeutic drug monitoring: voriconazole and posaconazole

    i)   Voriconazole: should be around 1.0~2.2 mg/L, caution when >6 mg/L

    ii) Posaconazole: >0.5~0.7 mg/L for prophylaxis, >1.8 mg/L for treatment

    iii) Close monitoring of CNI levels is recommended upon initiation, dose change, and discontinuation of azoles (strong, moderate).

    iv) Trough levels should be checked for voriconazole within 3-5 days and for posaconazole within 7 days of initiation, dose change, or change in clinical status that may affect drug levels (gut absorption, drug interactions) (strong, moderate).

(3) Pneumocystis jiroveci infection (Fishman et al., Clin Transplant, 33(9), e13587,2019)

  ① Risk factors for P. jiroveci infection

    i)   low total and CD4+ lymphocyte counts

    ii) CMV infection

    iii) Hypogammaglobulinemia

    iv) Graft rejection

    v) Patient age

  ② Diagnostic evaluation

i) Radiology

    (i) CXR: diffuse interstitial infiltrates

    (ii) Chest CT: GGO, reticular opacities, septal thickening, pneumatoceles

ii) Diagnostic specimen

    (i) BAL: Allows detection of multiple etiologies, yield $\geq$ 80% (Strong, high)

    (ii) Induced sputum: Alternative to BAL, yield $\geq$50% (Strong, high)

    (iii) Transbronchial biopsy: Increases yield of BAL, other lung pathology (Strong, moderate)

    (iv) Lung biopsy: Gold standard for diagnosis, generally not required (Strong, low)

iii) Diagnostic technique

    (i) Direct visualization of specimens using immunofluorescence assays: Most sensitive microscopic diagnostic method (Strong, high)

    (ii) Real-time qPCR, nucleic acid testing: Quantification in BAL; cannot distinguish infection from carriage (Strong, low)

    (iii) Silver, polychrome, or calcofluor stains: Exclusion of PJP by negative BAL only (Strong, high)

iv) Serum: may be inadequate due to low Ab production in transplant recipients and low sensitivity in acute disease.

    (i) β-d-glucan: Not specific, useful as adjunctive diagnostic tool; β-d-Glucan is component of P jiroveci cell wall (weak, moderate)High sensitivity (>90%) with lower specificity (<80%) and poor tracking with disease resolution. However, the $(1 \rightarrow 3)$ β-d-glucan assay has a high negative predictive value

(ii) LDH: Not specific, generally positive in PJP (Weak, low)

(iii) Genotyping, sequencing: Investigation of suspected outbreaks (Strong, low)

- Recommendations
    (i) Nonspecific indicators are useful including hypoxia, serum LDH, and β-d-glucan, which carry a high negative predictive value (strong, low).

    (ii) Nucleic acid amplification (NAT) may be useful but low specificity. Transplant patients with compatible syndromes and positive, validated NAT are likely to have PJP (strong, low).

    (iii) A definitive diagnosis of PJP is made by demonstration of organisms in lung tissue or respiratory tract secretions

    (iv) Initial diagnosis should be attempted using induced sputum examination coupled with direct immunofluorescent staining for P jiroveci (strong, moderate).

    (v) Invasive diagnosis should be considered if induced sputum not feasible (as is the case in younger children) or unrevealing and in transplant recipients with pneumonia without a microbiological diagnosis (strong, moderate).

(vi) Comment〉〉 이식환자에서의 PJP는 mortality/morbildity 가 높고, 치료 이후에도 lung tissue의 fibrosis및 emphysematous change를 남기므로 예방에 더불어 빠른 진단 및 치료가 중요함. 이식환자가 원인불명의 발열이 있는 경우 CXR상에서 GGO가 slowly progression하지는 않는지 주의 깊게 관찰하고 필요 시 non-contrast CT 촬영이 필요함. Chest CT상 bilateral GGO가 관찰될 경우 Infectious BAL/TBLB를 고려하고, BAL시행이 어려울 경우 Induced sputum 검체를 획득하여 PJP smear 및 PCR 검사의뢰 필요. PJP는 환자간 전염이 가능하므로 Induced sputum 획득 시에는 처치실 등 독립된 공간에서 시행. 장기간의 치료가 필요하므로 PJP smear로 확진이 필요하나 임상 경과에 따라 경험적 치료를 바로 고려해야 할 수 있으며 hypoxemia가 동반된 경우 adjunctive steroid투약이 필요함.

③ Therapeutic options

i) TMP-SMX: First line and drug of choice (Strong, high)

ii) Pentamidine: Second line in severe infection. Possible toxicities such as pancreatitis, hypo- and hyperglycemia, bone marrow suppression, renal failure, and electrolyte disturbances (Strong high)

iii) Other options: Atovaquone, Primaquine and clindamycin, Dapsone and trimethoprim, Macrolide and SMX, Caspofungin and TMP-SMX

iv) Adjunctives: Corticosteroids are best administered within 72 hours of presentation in the setting of hypoxia($PaO_2 \langle 70$ mmHg)

v) Duration of antimicrobials: at least 14 days (Strong, low)

vi) Comment〉〉 First line에 failure로 생각되는 경우에는 Second line agent로 Pentamidine 또는 Clindamycin + primaquine 으로 변경을 고려할 수 있으며, 그 외 약제는 국내에서 사용이 제한적임. 일반적으로 3주 치료를 시행하며 Adjunctive steroid 를 사용할 경우 recommended regimen (Pd 40 mg bid 5 days, 40 mg qd 5 days, 20 mg qd 11 days)이 있으나 HIV patient에서 evaluation된 regimen으로 non-HIV patient에서 는 임상경과에 맞추어 tapering을 결정함.

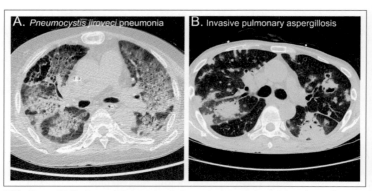

그림. Chest CT findings of Pneumocystis jiroveci pneumonia and invasive pulmonary aspergillosis

(4) Aspergillus infection

Inhalation is the most common route. A fumigatus is the most common species isolated (73%) Most cases (74%-78%) of invasive aspergillosis (IA) are limited to the lungs.

① Risk factors

 i) LT-early (0-3 months)

  (i) Re-transplantation (30-fold↑)

  (ii) Renal failure, RRT (25-fold↑)

  (iii) Fulminant hepatic failure

  (iv) MELD>30

  (v) Reoperation involving thoracic or intraabdominal cavity

 ii) LT-late (>3 months)

  (i) CMV infection (6-fold↑)

  (ii) Creatinine >3.3 g/dL

 iii) KT

  (i) Pre-transplant diagnosed COPD

  (ii) Acute rejection episode in last 3 months

  (iii) Graft failure

  (iv) High and prolonged duration of corticosteroid

② Clinical presentation

 i) Time of onset: Early in LT and HT compared to KT and lung T.

 ii) Symptoms: range from asymptomatic colonization to invasive presentations including sinusitis, tracheobronchitis, Invasive pulmonary aspergillosis (IPA), and empyema.

iii) Sites beyond respiratory system: mediastinitis, the musculoskeletal system, thyroid, skin, rhinocerebral disease, ocular, organ specific, endocarditis, central nervous system (CNS), and disseminated disease forms.

- LT is at high risk for dissemination and CNS involvement

iv) Prognosis: 3-month survival was 78% (Steinbach et al., J Infect. 2012;65(5):453-464.)

③ Diagnosis

i) CT: GGO (50%), peri-bronchial or mass-like consolidation (72%), macronodules. (59%) The "classic" halo sign and air-crescent signs are uncommon in SOT.

ii) Serum galactomannan (GM): not recommended to diagnose IA in SOT (Strong, moderate)

iii) BAL GM: preferred for the diagnosis of IPA in SOT (Strong; high)

iv) BAL GM index value cutoff of ≥ 1.0 is preferred for the diagnosis of IA in lung and non-lung transplant recipients, in combination with other fungal diagnostic modalities (eg, chest CT scan, culture) (Strong; moderate)

v) Standardized BAL Aspergillus PCR can be used in combination with other fungal diagnostic modalities (eg, chest CT scan, BAL GM, culture) for the diagnosis of IA. (Strong; low)

vi) Serum or BAL β-D-Glucan: not recommended for early screening and diagnosis of IA in lung T and LT recipients

(Strong; low)

④ Treatment recommendations (Supplement)

   i)   Early initiation of antifungals for strongly suspected patients is warranted (Strong, high)

   ii) Choice of antifungals

       (i)   Voriconazole is the drug of choice (Strong, high)

       (ii) Isavuconazole and lipid formulations of Amphotericin B (AmB), preferabley L-AmB can be alternative (Strong, moderate)

       (iii) Posaconazole can be a salvage therapy for treatment failure or intolerance to firt line antifungals (Strong, low)

       (iv) Although primary therapy with echinocandin is not recommended, (Strong, low) echinocandins can be considered when others are contraindicated (weak, low)

       (v) Combinations can be considered in selected cases with disseminated or CNS disease (weak, low)

   iii) Duration: guided by clinical and radiological response. Most cases will require minimum of 12 weeks (Strong, moderate)

   iv) Other recommendations

       (i)   Secondary prophylaxis: considered in patients with history of IA who undergo immunosuppression↑ and during prolonged neutropenia (<500/uL longer than 7 days) (weak, low)

       (ii) TDM: voriconazole (Strong, moderate)

    (iii) Drug interaction: dose of CNI/mTORi should be adjusted and monitored when starting and completing triazole therapy. (Supplement)

    (iv) Adverse effect: Baseline and follow-up ECG to assess QT interval (triazoles other than isavuconazole) and regular skin exam (voriconazole) are indicated for chronic azole therapy (Strong, high)

    (v) Surgery and reduction of immunosuppression are important adjunctive component (Strong, low)

    (vi) Colony-stimulating factors (e.g., G-CSF) may be considered in neutropenia (Strong, low)

⑤ Prevention

  i) General measure: exposure to Aspergillus ↓

    (i) 이식환자는 정원가꾸기, 밭농사, 가을에 낙엽쓸기 등을 하지 말아야하며 피할 수 없는 경우 반드시 마스크와 장갑을 착용해야 하며 신발/부츠, 긴바지, 긴팔옷 등을 입어야 함.

    (ii) 공사장이나 철거 현장에서는 반드시 N95마스크를 착용해야함.

    (iii) 흙이나 먼지에 노출된 이후에는 반드시 손을 씻어야 함.

  ii) Targeted prophylaxis for LT (Strong, moderate)

    (i) Re-transplantation (2nd or 3rd LT)

    (ii) RRT at the time of or within 7 days of transplantation

    (iii) Reopration involving thoracic or intra-abdominal cavity

  iii) Anidulafungin, micafungin or caspofungin in standard dose, or voriconazole is recommended for targeted prophylaxis in LT. (Strong, high)

iv) Targeted prophylaxis with a lipid formulation of amphotericin B (3-5 mg/kg) can be considered (weak, moderate)

v) Targeted prophylaxis should be continued for 14-21 days (Strong, high)

vi) Screening with serum GM and β-D-Glucan is not recommended for preemptive therapy (weak, low)

3) Viral infection

(1) CMV

① Definition

i) CMV infection

: Replicative infection diagnosed by intra-cytoplasmic or intra-nuclear inclusions or by antibody-based staining technique

ii) CMV syndrome

: Evidence of CMV in blood by viral culture, antigenemia or a DNA/RNA-based assay

: Plus One or more of the following

(i) Fever >38 ℃ for at least 2 days

(ii) New or increased malaise

(iii) Leukopenia

(iv) ≥5% atypical lymphocytes

(v) Thrombocytopenia

(vi) Elevation of hepatic transaminases (ALT or AST) to 2 × upper limit of normal (applicable to non-liver transplant recipients)

   iii) Tissue proven CMV disease

     : defined by evidence of CMV with pathology

② CMV antigenemia

   i) During the first month post-transplant: Proceed test on every Monday.

   → Proceed test on every Mon. Wed. Fri., if CMV antigenemia has a positive result.

   ii) During 1-3 months post-transplant: once a month

   iii) After 3 months (12 weeks): no routine follow up

③ Universal Prophylaxis

   i) CMV Donor IgG (+) / Recipient IgG (-)

     : IV ganciclovir 5 mg/kg iv q24h iv (normal renal function) prophylaxis during the hospital stay. Valganciclovir 900 mg (1T) qd (until POD#200 for KT, POD#100 for LT and other oragns)

     : If CMV antigenemia value becomes > 5/200,000 (in LT)/25/200,000 (in KT), switch to preemptive therapy (increased dosage: 5 mg/kg iv q12hr)

   ii) ATG, SPT (in pediatric) : IV ganciclovir prophylaxis

④ In KT recipients, prophylactic IV Ganciclovir is used for two weeks only in recipients with ATG induction.

⑤ Preemptive therapy

   i) CMV antigenemia

     a. > 5/200,000 (in LT)

     b. > 25/200,000 (in KT)

ii) Ganciclovir (IV) 5 mg/kg iv q12hr (normal renal function)
      until the CMV antigenemia value becomes zero, then stop

iii) Valganciclovir (Valcyte®) 2T (900 mg) bid for preemptive
      therapy
      until the CMV antigenemia value becomes zero, then stop

iv) In pediatric KT, only the CMV high-risk patient medicate
      valacyclovir.

⑥ Treatment of established CMV disease

i)   Ganciclovir 5 mg/kg q12hr iv for 2~6 weeks (at least 2
      weeks)

ii) F/U CMV disease: EGD, Sigmoidoscopy or colonoscopy,
      Biopsy

 -   CMV disease의 treatment response는 환자마다 상이하고 장
      기간의 치료를 요하는 경우가 많기 때문에 disease status에 대
      한 f/u이 필요하다

iii) Other agents: ganciclovir-resistant CMV → Foscarnet

iv) Renal impairment adjustment

Ganciclovir (DHPG)				
CCr	Dose	Dosing Interval	maintenance dose	dosing interval
(mL/min)	(mg/kg)	(hrs)	(mg/kg)	(hrs)
>70	5	12	5.0	24
50-69	2.5	12	2.5	24
25-49	2.5	24	1.25	24
10-24	1.25	24	0.625	24
<10 (intermittent HD)	1.25	3/wk after RRT	0.625	3/wk after RRT
CRRT	2.5	24	As above	As above

v) granulocyte $<1,000/mm^3$ or platelet $<20,000/mm^3$:
discontinue ganciclovir

	Proven or definite		Probable
CMV syndrome	Not defined	Detection of CMV in the blood by viral isolation, rapid culture, antigenemia, or QNAT Plus, at least two of the following: 1. Fever $\geq$38°C for at least 2 d 2. New or increased malaise or fatigue 3. Leukopenia or neutropenia on 2 separate measurements 4. 5% atypical lymphocytes 5. Thrombocytopenia 6. Hepatic aminotransferases increase to two times ULN (non-liver transplant recipients)	
Gastrointestinal CMV disease	Presence of upper and/ or lower GI symptoms plus macroscopic mucosal lesions plus CMV documented in tissue by histopathology, virus isolation, rapid culture, immunohistochemistry, or DNA hybridization techniques		Presence of upper and/or lower GI symptoms and CMV documented in tissue but without macroscopic mucosal lesions CMV documented in blood by NAT or antigenemia alone is not sufficient for diagnosis of CMV GI disease
CMV pneumonia	Clinical symptoms and/or signs of pneumonia such as new infiltrates on imaging, hypoxia, tachypnea, and/ or dyspnea combined with CMV documented in lung tissue by virus isolation, rapid culture, histopathology, immunohistochemistry, or DNA hybridization techniques		Clinical symptoms and/ or signs of pneumonia such as new infiltrates on imaging, hypoxia, tachypnea, and/or dyspnea combined with detection of CMV by viral isolation and rapid culture of BALF, or quantitation of CMV DNA in BALF

CMV hepatitis	Abnormal liver tests plus CMV documented in liver tissue by histopathology, IHC, virus isolation, rapid culture, or DNA hybridization techniques plus the absence of other documented cause of hepatitis	Not defined
CMV retinitis	Typical ophthalmological signs as assessed by an ophthalmologist experienced with the diagnosis of CMV Retinitis. If the presentation is atypical or an experienced ophthalmologist is not available, the diagnosis should be supported by CMV documented in vitreous fluid by NAT	Not defined
CMV encephalitis	CNS symptoms plus detection of CMV in CNS tissue by virus isolation, rapid culture, immunohistochemical analysis, in situ hybridization, or quantitative NAT	CNS symptoms plus detection of CMV in CSF without visible contamination of blood ("bloody tap") plus abnormal imaging results
Refractory CMV infection	CMV DNAemia or antigenemia increases (ie, >1 log10 increase in CMV DNA levels in blood between peak viral load within the first week and the peak viral load at 2 weeks or more) after at least 2 wk of appropriately dosed antiviral therapy	Viral load persistence (at the same level or higher than the peak viral load within 1 wk but <1 log10 increase in CMV DNA titers) after at least 2 wk of appropriately dosed antiviral therapy

Refractory CMV disease	Worsening in signs and symptoms or progression into end-organ disease after at least 2 wk of appropriately dosed antiviral therapy	Lack of improvement in clinical signs and symptoms after at least 2 wk of appropriately dosed antiviral therapy
Resistant CMV	Presence of viral genetic alteration that confer reduced susceptibility to one or more antiviral drugs	

Razonable et al., Clin Transplant , 33 (9), e13512 Sep 2019

(2) EBV

  ① No Prophylaxis

  ② Pre-emptive in high-risk recipients

    i) Ganciclovir (IV) for POD 2 wks and then acyclovir (PO) for 2 years

    ii) High-risk patients

      (i) Transplant from EBV IgG (+) donor to EBV IgG (-) recipient

      (ii) All children < 1 yr regardless of pretransplant serology

  ③ Acyclovir Dose

    i) Adult - 200 mg q 4 hr (5 times): 2 years old of older

    ii) Child - 100 mg q 4 hr (5 times) : under 2 years

  ④ PTLD (posttransplant lymphoproliferative disorder)

    i) Risk factors of PTLD

      (i) The patient on immune suppressant medication such as ATG.

      (ii) EBV D+/R- status

(iii) Fewer HLA matching

(iv) CMV D+/R- and CMV disease

(v) An aggressive work up is needed if the patient with risk factor has symptoms like fever, lymphadenopathy, diarrhea, allograft dysfunction.

ii) Diagnosis and management of PTLD

    (i) P/E for cervical/axillary/inguinal LN enlargement

    (ii) Abdomen US or CT for detection of LN enlargement

    (iii) Mucosa biopsy via sigmoidoscopy (colonoscopy)

    (iv) LN biopsy, if palpable or enlarged

    (v) Tonsillectomy (biopsy)

    (vi) Reduction of immunosuppression

-   $\downarrow$ cyclosporine/tacrolimus to $\frac{1}{2}$ or less

-   Stop azathioprine/MMF

-   Maintain oral steroid

-   Time to response; 2-4 wks

    (vii) Anti-CD20 antibodies (Rituximab - 375 mg/m^2)

-   Neutralizing the B-cells expressing CD20

-   Abort the lytic-replicative phase of EBV-driven lymphoproliferation

iii) A high EBV DNA load (EBV PCR > 2000 copies/5μL whole blood) in the peripheral blood is associated with an increased risk on PTLD.

    (i) Reduction of immunosuppression

    (ii) Antiviral medication ± IVIG

    (iii) Monoclonal B-cell antibody therapy

(iv) Surgical resection

iv) Baseline study in pediatric LT: EBV PCR

Preop~Postop 1yr	Every 1 month
~Postop 2yr	q 2 months
~after 2yr	q 4 months

(3) VZV, HSV

① No prophylaxis

② Treatment for Herpes infection

: Acyclovir 10-14 days

③ Dose of Intravenous Acyclovir

CCr (mL/min)	Induction Dose (mg/kg)	Dosing Interval (hrs)
>50	10	8
25-50	10	12
10-24	10	24
<10	5	24

④ Dose of Oral Acyclovir

CCr (mL/min)	Induction Dose (mg/kg)	Dosing Interval (hrs)
>50	800 mg	6
10-50	800 mg	8
<10	800 mg	24

(4) HBV infection in LT

① HBV Prophylaxis in HBsAg (+) recipient : HBIG + entecavir p.o.

i) Hepabig 10,000U (in pediatric patient; 100 IU/kg(under 30 kg), 10,000U (30 kg or over)) ivs + 5%DW 200 cc mix IV

i) In case preoperative HBV-DNA or HBeAg of recipient is

positive; inject Hepabig 20,000 U (until post-transplant 4 weeks)

ii) Give the first dose at an anhepatic phase intra-operatively. Inject once daily until POD#6 (7th dose). Then, 1 inj/ wk for the next 3 weeks. (Give 10 times during the first month) Give 10,000U ivs every month until 1year after transplant.

iii) Give once monthly or every other month according to HBs-Ab titer, after 1year of transplant. (cut-off value; HBsAb titer > 200)

v) If the recipient has no history of antiviral agent medication before liver transplantation: Start Entecavir (dose: 0.5 mg qd) at POD #1.

vi) If the recipient has a history of antiviral agent medication before liver transplantation, do the following:

(i) Keep the same antiviral agent used before liver transplantation.

(ii) A confirmation of attending is needed if the patient has trouble in renal function.

CCr (mL/min)	Dose (entecavir)
≥50	Once daily 0.5 mg
30–<50	Once daily 0.25 mg or 0.5 mg q 48hrs
10–<30	Once daily 0.15 mg or 0.5 mg q 72hrs
<10, HD or CAPD	Once daily 0.05 mg or 0.5 mg q 7 days

vii) If patient get negative conversion of HBV (previously (+), latterly (-)), start Entecavir 0.5 mg qd only (without HBIG)

② De novo hepatitis B prophylaxis in HBcAb (+) donor

   i) Hepabig 10,000U (pediatric; 100 IU/kg) ivs + 5%DW 100 cc mix IV

   ii) Give the first dose at anhepatic phase intraoperatively, inject once daily until POD#6 (7th dose).

   iii) Keep HBs-Ab titer > 200 after the first week. (HBIG 10,000 U (adult)/ 2,000 U IV (pediatric) IVS)

   iv) Change to the active vaccination (Hepavax, Euvax), in pediatric patients, after 1year. (keep HBs-Ab titer 100 or over)

③ Treatment of Recurrent HBV

   i) If the patient's HBsAg converted to positive result on routine follow-up

   ii) Hepatitis profile check, HBV DNA quantitation, HBV YMDD mutation check

   iii) Start Entecavir: 0.5 mg qd

CCr (mL/min)	Dose	lamivudine resistance (+) Dose
≥ 50	Once daily 0.5 mg	Once daily 1 mg
30-50	once daily 0.25 mg or 0.5 mg/48hrs	once daily 0.5 mg or 1 mg/48hrs
10-30	once daily 0.15 mg or 0.5 mg/72hrs	once daily 0.3 mg or 1 mg/72hrs
<10, HD[a] or CAPD	once daily 0.05 mg or 0.5 mg/7days	once daily 0.1 mg or 1 mg/7days

[a] r 1mg/7days. 1mg check it is given on HD day.

④ Pediatric patients without HBcAb (+) group (including HBsAg

(-) child)

  : Proceed Hepatitis profile routine follow up every 6mo. keep HBs-Ab titer more than 10.

(5) HBsAg (+) in Kidney recipient

  : Post-transplant → hepatologist consult (Anti-viral agent start)

(6) HCV infection in LT

  ① Preoperative management

    i)   Check HCV genotype, HCV RNA titer

    ii) History of IFN or ribavirin treatment

    iii) IL28B genotype (CC, TT, or TC)

  ② Postoperative management

    i)   Check HCV RNA

       (i)   2 weeks, 1, 3, 6 months, then annually

       (ii) Typically, HCV RNA levels increase rapidly on post-op week 2, peaking at 4 months.

       (iii) At 1 year, HCV RNA levels are usually 10-20 times greater than pretransplant levels.

    ii) Protocol biopsy

       (i)   1 year after LT

       (ii) Annual biopsy

    iii) Anti-rejection therapy

       (i)   Increase CNI or MMF dosage

       (ii) Steroid pulse therapy is considered when,

       -   Moderate~severe rejection

       -   No response after 1 week of CNI/MMF elevation

  ③ Antiviral therapy for Hepatitis C

i) All patients with HCV recurrence should be treated.

ii) Medication

    (i) PEG-interferon + ribavirin combination therapy: very limited in use because of the side effect and rejection.

    (ii) Oral medication (DAA, direct antiviral agents) combination therapy: Most transplant patient can use safely.

iii) Classification of oral medication

    (i) NS3/4A protease inhibitor (asunaprevir, simeprevir, etc. they end with -evir)

    (ii) NS5A inhibitor (daclatasvir, ledipasvir, etc. they end with -avir)

    (iii) NS5B NUC inhibitor (sofosbuvir, it ends with -uvir)

    (iv) NS5B non-NUC inhibitor (dasabuvir, it ends with -uvir)

iv) Characteristics of oral medication

    (i) If you do not combine the medications, treatment fails because of mutation. - Combine drugs with a different mechanism.

    (ii) Complicated Drug-drug interaction. Be cautious, a dose of the immune suppressant during the treatment. A Severe side effect could be accrued including arrhythmia, heart failure, etc. It is rare, but it can happen.

    (iii) Depending on the genotype of the HCV, some drugs work and others not. The combination of drugs should be chosen according to the genotype.

④ Risk factors for more severe recurrence of HCV (Strengh of evidence)

   i)   Donor age (+++)

   ii) Living donor (+)

   iii) Donor/recipient HLA matching (+)

   iv) Genotype 1B (+)

   v) HIV coinfection (+++)

   vi) Longer CIT (++)

   vii) Donor genetic factors (+)

   viii)Recipient age (+++)

   ix) Higher pretransplant viral load (+++)

   x) Higher posttransplant viral load (+++)

   xi) Steroid pulse therapy (+++)

   xii) Short time to recurrence (+++)

   xiii) Treated CMV infection (+++)

(7) Polyomavirus (BK virus) - KT

   ① tubulointerstitial nephritis

   ② screening and monitoring for unexplained serum creatinine elevation

   ③ Algorithm for the screening, management, and monitoring of patient with BKVAN

**Urine BK virus DNA PCR detection at
POD #1, 5, 9, 16, 24, 36, 48 weeks**

if positive

Check urine BK virus DNA PCR quantitation

if urine BK DNA viral load ≥ 7 log copies/ml

Check plasma BK virus DNA PCR quantitation

if serum BK DNA viral load ≥ 4 log copies/ml
with creatinine elevation, or clinically suspects

Allograft biopsy

If the Urine BK test result is over 7 log copies, stop MMF and proceed serum BK test!!!

4) Latent Tuberculosis treatment

   (1) Pre-transplantation w/u에서 TB Specific Interferon-Gamma결과
      가 양성이고, Chest CT상에서 Old TB lesion이 있거나 불충분한 결
      핵 치료력이 있는 경우 고려

   (2) Donor Quantiferon (+)/Recipient Quantiferon (-) 인 경우 고려

   (3) 이식 후 결핵에 노출된 경우 고려

   (4) Regimen: INH 300 mg (9개월) + B6 50 mg

3. Fever in the transplant recipients

   1) Fever without localizing findings

      (1) Chest PA

      (2) Blood culture

      (3) U/A and Urine Culture

(4) CMV antigenemia

2) Pneumonia: R/O

   (1) Chest PA

   (2) Blood culture

   (3) Sputum Gram stain and culture (including fungus)

   (4) Sputum AFB smear and culture

   (5) Sputum respiratory virus panel (multiplex PCR)

   (6) Pneumococcus and Legionella urinary antigen

   (7) M. pneumoniae antibody & IgM

   (8) Influenza antigen (nasopharyngeal swab; 유행 시)

   (9) CMV antigenemia

   (10) Aspergillosis Ag

   (11) Consider HRCT

   (12) Consider Bronchoscopy with BAL (bacterial, viral, AFB and fungal culture; PCR for P. jirovecii, CMV, respiratory virus panel; Aspergillus Ag when IPA is suspected)

   (13) Consider Anti-fungal agent administration if not improved with antibiotics

3) UTI (for kidney transplant recipient)

   (1) Urine Gram stain and culture

   (2) Blood Gram stain and culture

   (3) Consider VCUG, if recurrent: R/O Reflex

4) Cholangitis (for liver transplant recipient)

   (1) Blood and Bile Gram stain and culture

   (2) Doppler US or Liver CT: R/O Biliary complications

   (3) Consider intervention - PTBD, PCD, ERCP

5) Diarrhea

   (1) Stool culture (Salmonella, Shigella, Campylobacter)

   (2) Stool exam: Parasite, Protozoa (cryptosporidium, microsporidium)

   (3) Clostridium difficile toxin

   (4) CMV antigenemia : R/O CMV enteritis

   (5) Consider sigmoidoscopy in prolonged and severe diarrhea

   (6) Abdomen-Pelvis CT: R/O PTLD

   (7) Common Causes of Diarrhea after LT (Ordered as frequency

      ① ++++: CMV, C.diff, MMF

      ② +++: Cyclosporine, tacrolimus, sirolimus

      ③ ++: IBD

      ④ +: Campylobacter, adenovirus astrovirus, rotavirus, salmonella, lactose intolerance, GVHD, PTLD, colon cancer, villous adenoma, celiac sprue, microsporidia, cryptosporidia, shigella, amoebiasis, bacterial overgrowth.

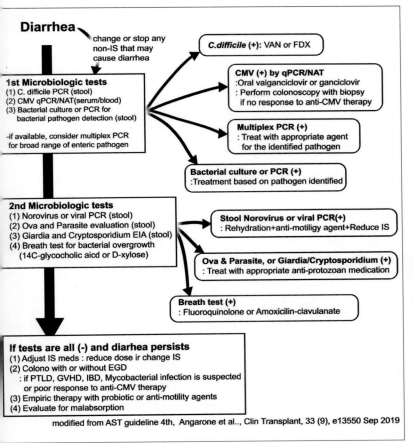

Diarrhea
→ change or stop any non-IS that may cause diarrhea

1st Microbiologic tests
(1) C. difficile PCR (stool)
(2) CMV qPCR/NAT(serum/blood)
(3) Bacterial culture or PCR for bacterial pathogen detection (stool)

-if available, consider multiplex PCR for broad range of enteric pathogen

C.difficile (+): VAN or FDX

CMV (+) by qPCR/NAT
:Oral valganciclovir or ganciclovir
: Perform colonoscopy with biopsy if no response to anti-CMV therapy

Multiplex PCR (+)
: Treat with appropriate agent for the identified pathogen

Bacterial culture or PCR (+)
:Treatment based on pathogen identified

2nd Microbiologic tests
(1) Norovirus or viral PCR (stool)
(2) Ova and Parasite evaluation (stool)
(3) Giardia and Cryptosporidium EIA (stool)
(4) Breath test for bacterial overgrowth (14C-glycocholic aicd or D-xylose)

Stool Norovirus or viral PCR(+)
: Rehydration+anti-motiligy agent+Reduce IS

Ova & Parasite, or Giardia/Cryptosporidium (+)
: Treat with appropriate anti-protozoan medication

Breath test (+)
: Fluoroquinolone or Amoxicilin-clavulanate

If tests are all (-) and diarrhea persists
(1) Adjust IS meds : reduce dose ir change IS
(2) Colono with or without EGD
: if PTLD, GVHD, IBD, Mycobacterial infection is suspected or poor response to anti-CMV therapy
(3) Empiric therapy with probiotic or anti-motility agents
(4) Evaluate for malabsorption

modified from AST guideline 4th, Angarone et al.., Clin Transplant, 33 (9), e13550 Sep 2019

그림. 이식환자에서 설사 work-up guideline

* Graft versus Host Disease (GVHD) after LT (Murali et al.,
  Transplantation 2016.Dec;100(12): 2661-2670)

  (1) Introduction

    ① Rare but extremely severe complication after organ
      transplantation

    ② Median time to GVHD onset is 28days

  (2) Diagnosis

    ① Sx : Skin rash (92%), Pancytopenia (78%), diarrhea (65%)

    ② Pathologic Dx : Skin, colonoscopy or bone marrow.
      Confirmation : short tandem repeat (STR) test for CD3+ donor
      lymphocytes

  (3) Treatment

    ① No Specific treatment is confirmed to improve survival

    ② TNF alpha inhibitor (Etanercept or infliximab) showed case
      report of effectiveness

  (4) Conclusion

    ① Early suspicion & diagnosis is very important

    ② Treatment must be confirmed by professor.

      (Acute Graft-versus-host disease after liver transplant: Novel
      Use of Etanercept and the role of tumor necrosis factor α
      inhibitors. Liver transplantation 15:421-426, 200))

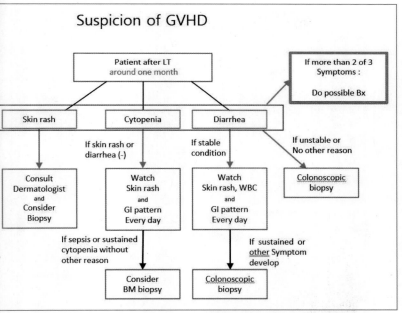

그림. 이식환자에서 GVHD 의심 시 SMC work-up flow

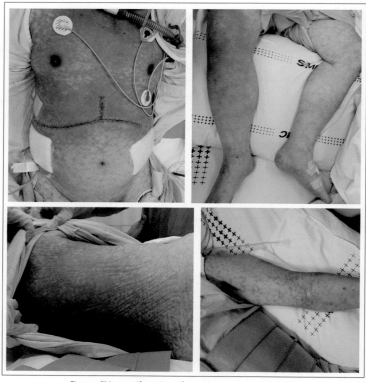

Figure. Skin manifestation of maculopapular rash in GVHD patient after LT

CHAPTER 04.

DECEASED DONOR EVALUATION AND MANAGEMENT

I. Donor criteria

1. 뇌사자에서 장기별 특정 선정/제외 기준

1) General Exclusion Criteria

(1) Evidence of HIV or active hepatitis B infection

(2) Presence of history of extracranial malignancy

(3) Severe systemic sepsis

(4) Disease of unknown etiology

2) Kidney

(1) Acceptable Criteria

① No evidence of primary renal diseases

② No history of long-standing hypertension or diabetes

③ Normal urinalysis

④ Urine output > 0.5 mL/kg/hr

⑤ Normal BUN and Creatinine

(2) Ideal Donor Criteria

① Age 10-39 years old

② Cause of Death: No cerebrovascular disease

③ Creatinine ≤1.5 mg/dL

3) Liver

(1) Acceptable Criteria

① Age≤60 years

② No evidence of active hepatitis

③ No upper limit of AST/ALT

4) Pancreas

(1) Acceptable Criteria

① Age 10-45 years

② No history of DM

③ No history of chronic pancreatitis

④ No upper limit of serum amylase

(2) Relative Contraindications

① Gross obesity: BMI > 30 kg/m²

② Peripheral vascular disease

③ Ischemic heart disease

5) Heart

(1) Acceptable Criteria

① < 55 years old

② Heart disease가 없는 경우

(2) Relative Contraindication

   ① MI가 있는 경우

   ② Moderate이상의 Valve disease가 있는 경우

   ③ A.fib

   ④ Cardiomyopathy

   ⑤ 60세 이상

   ⑥ Cold ischemic time이 4-5시간 이상인 경우

   ⑦ Coronary disease (one or two vessel disease)

6) Lung

  (1) Ideal donor lung selection criteria

   ① Age less than 55 years

   ② ABO blood group compatible, donation-after-brain death lung

   ③ Appropriate size match

   ④ Clear chest radiograph

   ⑤ PaO_2/FiO_2 >300 on FiO_2 of 100%, PEEP of 5 cmH_2O

   ⑥ History of tobacco use less than 20 pack-years

   ⑦ Absence of chest trauma

   ⑧ No evidence of aspiration or sepsis

   ⑨ Absence of purulent secretions at bronchoscopy

   ⑩ Absence of organisms on sputum Gram stain

   ⑪ No history of primary pulmonary disease or active pulmonary infection

  (2) Acceptable donor lung selection criteria (extended donor criteria)

   ① Age less than 70 years

② Compatible ABO blood group for brain death or cardiac death donors

③ Approximate size match, with minor surgical trimming or lobectomy as needed

④ Minor diffuse and moderate focal chest radiograph changes are acceptable if good, stable/improving function

⑤ PaO_2/FiO_2 >250 on FiO_2 of 100%, PEEP of 5 cmH_2O

⑥ History of tobacco use less than 40 pack years

⑦ Chest trauma is not relevant if good function

⑧ Aspiration or minor sepsis are acceptable if good, stable/improving function

⑨ Purulent secretions not relevant if good, stable/improving function

⑩ Organisms on Gram stain and ventilation time are not relevant

⑪ Primary pulmonary disease is not acceptable, except asthma

2. 뇌사자에서 장기별 marginal donor 기준(종류) 및 참고 지침 (KONOS 규정)

1) Kidney

(1) Age > 60 years

(2) Serum creatinine > 3.0 mg/dL or Creatinine Clearance < 60

(3) Kidney Marginal 이식대상자 선정기준

이식대상자 선정을 위한 매칭결과 상위 제 3순위인 자까지 매칭결과를 해당 기관에 통보하여도 이식대상자가 선정되지 아니하는 경

우 뇌사자를 관리하고 있는 뇌사판정대상자관리기관에 이식대상자
선정 우선권을 부여.

(4) 양쪽 신장을 모두 기증할 수 있는 조건 (하나 이상 만족시 해당)

   ① 나이가 3세 이하인 경우

   ② 체중이 15 kg 이하인 경우

   ③ Sono 검사상 신장크기가 6 cm 이하인 경우

   ④ 70세 이상이면서 다음 한 가지 이상 해당하는 경우

      i)   serum creatineine clearance (MDRD=GFR) < 30 mL

      ii)   serum creatine > 3.0 mg/dl

2) Liver (아래항목 3가지 이상 해당)

  (1) 최근 12시간 동안 강심제 사용여부 상관없이 SBP < 60 mmhg 1시
간 초과

  (2) 최근 12시간 동안 6시간 이상 강심제 사용.

    Dopamine > 15 μg /kg/min   or   Amines > 0.2 μg/kg/min

  (3) ICU day > 7day

  (4) Na^+ > 160 mEq/L 최근 검사 중 2회 이상 유지 (6시간 이상)

  (5) T- bil > 2.5 mg/dl 최근 검사 중 2회 이상 유지 (6시간 이상)

  (6) PT < 40% 최근 검사 중 2회 이상 유지 (6시간 이상)

    분할이식 기증자의 조건

   ① 혈동학적으로 안정되고 심장이 뛰고 있는 뇌사 상태의 다장기
기증자

   ② 연령이 40세 이하면서 체중이 50 kg 이상

   ③ 1차 뇌사조사 후 간장 이식대상자 선정 시점까지, 다음과 같은
기준의 혈압 상승약 사용이 모두 해당하는 경우

      i)   Dopamine 15 mg/kg/min 이하

      ii)   Dobutamine 15 mg/kg/min 이하

      iii) Norepinephrine 0.75 mg/kg/min 이하

      iv) Epinephrine 0.075 mg/kg/min 이하

④ 1차 뇌사 조사 이후 중환자실 재원일수 5일 이하인 경우 (참고)

⑤ 적출 당시 24시간 전에 OT/PT 검사결과가 정상의 3배 이하인 경우 (참고)

⑥ 적출 당시 24시간 전에 S-Na이 160 mg/dl 이하인 경우 (참고)

3. 뇌사자에서 장기별 특정 선정 검사 protocol

1) Routine General Examination

   (1) Laboratory Exam

     ① Blood: CBC, Chemistry profile (LFT, e', BUN/Cr), PT/aPTT, Direct-Bilirubin, ABGA, amylase/lipase, CK/CK-MB/LDH, Troponin, HbA1c

     ② Culture: Blood culture (peripheral 2 set, central line있을 경우 lumen별 1쌍), Gram stain and culture (urine, sputum), Fungus culture (sputum)

     ③ MDR pathogen screening: Nasal MRSA culture, VRE rectal screening, CRE screening (rectal swab), Carbapenemase gene PCR (rectal swab)

     ④ Urine: Urinalysis with micro, Urine- osm, Urine- creatine/ protein ratio, albumin/creatine ratio. Urine -e

     ⑤ Serologic assay: HBsAg, anti-HBs Ab, HBeAg, anti-HBe Ab, anti-HBc Ab (IgG/IgM), anti-HCV Ab, anti-HAV Ab (IgG/IgM), anti-HIV combo, RPR, TPLA, CMV Ab (IgG), EB-VCA (IgG), TB Specific Interferone-Gamma (QFT)

     ⑥ Radiologic Exam: Chest X-ray, LGPK US, 2D-echocardiography (heart donation 시), ((prn) Brain non-contrast CT)

(2) Radiologic Exam: Chest X-ray, abdomen sono, 2D-echocardiography (heart donation 시), Brain non-contrast CT (필요 시)

(3) Physiologic Exam: EKG, EEG, Broncoscopy (lung 선정팀 요청 시)

2) Kidney

  (1) Serum Bun & Creatinine

    * Cr < 3.0인 경우도 수일에 걸쳐 조금씩 계속 증가하는 경우 예후가 안 좋다.

  (2) Urine lab

  (3) abdomen sono

  (4) Kidney biopsy (Intraoperative)

3) Liver

  (1) Serum sample: Chemistry profile (LFT, e'), PT (INR), HBsAg, anti-HBs, anti-HBc (IgG/IgM), anti-HCV, anti-HAV (IgG/IgM),

    * Na+ > 155 mEq/L시 graft PNF risk가 증가한다는 보고가 있으므로 교정요함.

  (2) Abdomen sono

  (3) Intraoperative Frozen biopsy

4) Pancreas

  (1) Serum amylase/ lipase

  (2) HgA1c

  (3) Intraoperative inspection and palpation

5) Heart

  (1) 2-D echo, EKG

  (2) CK/CK-MB, Troponin

6) Lung

(1) Chest X-ray

(2) Bronchoscopy

(3) ABGA (PaO$_2$ / FiO$_2$ 100% & 40%)

(4) Sputum culture (TTA)

II. 뇌사판정 절차

1. Deceased donor 판정 및 harvest 전의 절차

시점	내용	Etc
ICU 입실	Ventilator setting	
	A-line, C-line, L-tube ins.	
	뇌사자 처방 1) 기본처방 2) 약물처방 3) 검사처방 ◇ Blood CBC, Chemistry profile (LFT, e', BUN/Cr), PT/aPTT, D-Bilirubin, ABGA, amylase/lipase, CK/CK-MB/LDH, Troponin, HgA1C, HLA typing ◇ Culture Blood(2쌍), Urine, Sputum Gram stain and culture (including fungus) Nasal- MRSA, rectal- VRE ◇ Urine Urinalysis with micro, Urine– osm, Urine- creatine/protein ratio, albumin/creatine ratio. Urine –e ◇ Selorogy HBsAg, anti-HBs, HBeAg, anti-HBe, anti-HBc (IgG/IgM), anti-HCV, anti-HAV (IgG/IgM), anti-HIV, CMV (IgG/IgM), EBV (IgG/IgM), VDRL, TPLA, ◇ Radiologic Exam Chest X-ray, Abdomen US, 2D-echocardiography (heart 기증 시), ((prn) Brain non-contrast CT) ◇ Physiologic Exam EKG, EEG, bronchoscopy (lung 기증 시)	혈액 sample 약 150 cc Sample후 Hgb, V/S obs.
	환자 상태 파악 및 약물조정 Target baseline : MAP > 75 mmHg, UO > 1 mL/kg/hr, P/F > 200 (lung donation 시 P/F > 300) 유지	Donor Mx protocol 참고

1차 조사	PCO₂ 35-45 mmHg, SBP 100 mmHg 이상, FiO₂ 100% 10분 이상 apply로 baseline 조정		
	1차조사 시행(뇌간검사(법률 별지에 항목 있음), apnea test) : apnea test fail시 TCD로 대체 (1-2차 간격:2개월-1세:48시간/1세- 6세:24시간/6세이상:6시간)		Apnea test 이후 환자 상태 close obs. (CO₂ retention, Acidosis)
장기 평가	Heart	2-D echo, EKG	선정 시 prn cardiac lab
	Lung	Chest X-ray, ABGA (bronchoscopy)	선정 시 prn O₂ full ABGA
	Liver	Abd-sono, S-lab	
	Pancreas	Abd-sono, HLA, S-lab	선정시 prn Amy/ lipase
	Kidney	Abd-sono, HLA, S-lab	
	Cornea	S-lab, 각막수술여부	Dura tear 처방
2차 조사	PCO₂ 35-45 mmHg, SBP 100 mmHg 이상, FiO₂ 100% 10분 이상 apply로 baseline 조정		
	2차조사 시행(뇌간검사(법률 별지에 항목 있음), apnea test) : apnea test fail시 TCD로 대체		Apnea test 이후 환자 상태 close obs. (CO₂ retention, Acidosis)
EEG	30분 이상의 평탄뇌파 확인		
뇌사판정 위원회	과반수이상 참석, 만장일치 시 통과. 종료시간: 사망시간		
검시전 적출 승인	병사의 경우는 생략		
Harvest OP	장기 선정 병원과 수술시간 조정		

2. Apnea test protocol(법에 기반한 SMC 규정)

(1) FiO₂ 1.0의 산소를 10분 이상 인공호흡기로 흡입시킨다.

(2) 검사 직전 Baseline ABGA를 실시한다(Baseline ABGA는 PaCO₂ 35~45 mmHg 정도로 설정한 : ETCO₂ monitor 를 이용하여 맞춘다).

(3) 100% O_2 6 L/min의 산소를 계속 공급한다.

(4) 검사 시작 후 환자 상태에 따라 10분 이내에 1~5분 간격으로 ABGA를 실시한다.

(5) $PaCO_2$가 50 mmHg 이상으로 상승하였음에도 불구하고 자발호흡이 관찰되지 않으면 자발호흡이 되살아날 수 없다고 판정하고 Apnea test 를 마친다.

(6) 만일 검사도중 SBP 70 mmHg 이하 또는 O_2saturation (on pulse oximeter) 90%이하 시 중지한다. - TCD 대체

III. Deceased Donor Management

1. Intensive monitoring and management at ICU

(1) Review all medications previously ordered

: Anti-convulsant, pain medication, osmotic agent are not necessary and should be discontinued.

(2) Vital sign and Hemodynamic monitoring & management

: 충분한 fluid resuscitation 중에도 저혈압이 지속되는 경우 최근에는 저용량의 vasopressin의 사용이 늘고 있다. Vasopressin 은 뇌사 후 발생하는 vasodilatory shock에 효과적이고 요붕증의 치료로 사용되며, 카테콜아민의 요구량을 줄여준다. 기타 norepinephrine, epinephrine, dobutamine, dopamine 등의 vasopressor, 혹은 inotropic agent가 혈역학적 유지를 위해 사용될 수 있다. Tachyarrhythmia가 동반된 경우 dopamine, dobutamine, epinephrine의 사용에 주의한다.

① Mean Arterial Pressure (MAP) via A-line ≥ 75 mmHg

일반적으로 뇌사자 관리 시 MAP 60~100 mmHg를 유지하는 것을 목표로 하나, 중환자관리 시 MAP를 높게 유지할 경우 급성신부전의

발생이 감소함을 참고하여 높은 목표치를 설정한다.

② Systolic Blood Pressure (SBP) ≤ 160~170 mmHg

- Standard inotropic or vasopressor support
    a. Arginine vasopressin 0.01~0.03 IU/min (max 0.04 IU/min)
    b. Norepinephrine 0.05~2.0 μg/kg/min
    c. Dopamine 5~10 μg/kg/min
    d. Epinephrine 0.05~0.15 μg/kg/min
    e. Thyroid hormone
- SBP >160 mmHg or MAP >90 mmHg인 경우 고혈압의 치료가 이루어져야 한다
    a. Tachycardia가 동반된 hypertension의 경우 primary choice는 short acting beta blocker인 Esmolol을 100-500 μg/kg bolus 투약 후 100-300 μg/kg/min CIV 적용.
    b. Labetalol 10 mg IV bolus q 20 min 또는 Nicardipine 5 mg/hr CIV
    c. Nitroprusside 0.5-5.0 μg/kg/min

③ Heart Rate (HR) 60~120 beats/min

④ Body Temperature (BT) > 34℃ (acidosis, arrhythmia, coagulopathy, bleeding tendency 등이 동반된 경우에는 36.5~37.8℃ normothermia target으로 warming 시행한다.)

: Warmed IV fluids, warming blanket, heated and humidified inspired gas

: 38℃ 이상의 고열이 발생할 경우 external cooling과 함께 bromocriptine 투여를 고려할 수 있다.

⑤ Urine output: 0.5~3 mL/kg/hr

⑥ Medication으로 적절히 유지되지 않는 LV failure의 경우 VA ECMO적용을 고려

(3) Pulmonary Artery Catheterization (PAC)

① Indication for PAC

- 심초음파상에 Ejection Fraction (EF) < 40%이거나
- 고용량의 dopamine (>10 μg/kg/min) 을 투약하거나
- Vasopressor를 쓰는 경우: 심박출량(Cardiac Output. CO), 체혈관 저항(systemic vascular resistance, SVR) 등을 측정하기 위해 폐동맥 도관 삽관을 고려할 수 있다.

② PAC hemodynamic target

- Pulmonary Capillary Wedge Pressure (PCWP) 6~10 mmHg
- Cardiac Index (CI) > 2.4 L/min/m2
- Systemic Vascular Resistance (SVR) 800-1200 dynes/s-cm5
- Left Ventricular stroke work index (LVSWI)>15 g/kg/min

③ 최근 CO, SV, SVV, SVR 등의 monitoring을 위해 PAC외에 semi-invasive device (EV-1000, PiCCO 등..) 사용이 늘고있다.

(4) Mechanical Ventilation

① Setting

- Tidal volume 6~8 mL/kg
- PEEP 5~8 cmH$_2$O
- Peak Inspiratory Pressure (PIP) ≤ 30cmH$_2$O
- P/F > 200

② PaCO$_2$ 35~45 mmhg유지한다. O$_2$ saturation > 95%

③ 폐 이식을 고려하는 경우 low tidal volume, FiO$_2$ < 60% 미만을 유지하며 PEEP을 10 cmH$_2$O으로 유지하고 P/F ratio 300 이상을 target으로 ventilator setting을 한다. High dose methylprednisolone [15 mg/kg (max. 1000 mg)] 정맥 투여를 고려할 수 있다.

(5) Head elevation: 약 30도 상승

(6) Frequent tracheal suction and position change

(7) Nasogastric tube의 유지 및 흡인

(8) Maintenance fluid therapy

: BP, U/O, e'에 따라 main fluid 종류 및 투여 속도 조절

(9) Fluid & Electrolyte management

혈청 포타슘은 3.5 mEq/L이하로 떨어지지 않도록 유지하여야 하고, 혈청 소디움은 130-150 mEq/L (> 160 mEq/L시 5% DW로), 소변량은 0.5~3 mL/hr으로 유지한다. 요붕증 치료의 목적은 저혈량을 교정하고 혈청 소디움을 정상수준으로 되돌리는데 있다. Low dose vasopressin infusion (0.01~0.03 IU/min, max 0.04 IU/min)은 소변량을 조절 가능한 수준으로 낮출 수 있다. 그러나 심한 경우 Desmopressin [1-D-amino-8-D-arginine vasopressin (DDAVP)]를 함께 투약하는 것이 필요하다.

① Diabetes Insipidus의 정의

- Urine output > 4 mL/kg per hr
- Associated with rising serum sodium (≥145 mmol/L)
- Associated with rising serum osmolarity (≥300 mOsm)
- Decreasing urine osmolarity (≤200 mOsm)

② Management of DI

- 저혈압이 동반된경우; Low-dose vasopressin infusion (0.01~0.03 IU/min, max 0.04 IU/min)
- Desmopressin (DDAVP)은 arginine vasopressin의 synthetic analogue로 비교적 순수한 항이뇨작용이 있으며 vasopressor

작용은 미약하다.

   a. 성인: 1-4 μg IV then 1-2 μg IV every 6 hr. 목표 소변량 < 4 mL/kg/h

   b. 소아: 0.25-1 μg IV every 6 hr. 목표소변량 < 4 mL/kg/h

(10) Hormone replace therapy

- Vasopressin: 뇌사자에서 바소프레신 결핍은 요붕증을 발생시킬 수 있으며, 요붕증의 진단기준에 맞지 않는 뇌사자라 하더라도 저혈압과 감소된 순환용적에 반응하는 baroreflex-mediated AVP 분비에 장애가 있어 혈관수축이 저하되어있다. 그러므로 vasopressin은 DI의 동반여부와 관련없이, 적절한 수액치료 후에도 저혈압이 지속되는경우 투여되어야 한다. (0.01~0.03 IU/min, max 0.04 IU/min)

- Corticosteroid: low dose hydrocortisone (hydrocortisone 300 mg/day) 투여가 vasopressor의 요구량을 감소시키고 순환부전의 회복에 도움이 된다. 폐기증이 예정된 경우 high-dose MPD 투여를 고려할 수 있다(MPD 15 mg/kg, max. 1000 mg).

- Thyroid hormone: 혈역학적 안정에 도움을 준다는 보고가 있어 투여 고려할 수 있으나, 국내에서는 IV 제제 사용 불가임. (T4 20 μg IV than 10 μg/hr CIV, or T3 4 μg IV than 3 μg/hr CIV)

(11) Glycemic control: ICU BST control protocol에 따라 140~180 mg/dL로 유지한다.

  : 혈당의 조절은 특히 췌장 & Islet cell 구득시에 중요한데, β-세포에 과도한 스트레스를 피하는 것이 좋다.

(12) Infection Control

감염의 의심병변에 맞추어 시작한다(모든 항생제 renal dose adjustment에 주의).

① Routine exam에 포함된 culture 및 serology 검사를 시행한다.

② 발열등의 감염을 시사하는 소견이 있거나 활력징후가 불안정 할 경우에는 Blood/sputum/urine culture를 반복한다.

③ 경험적인 광범위 항생제는 적응증이 아니며, 확인된 감염에 대해서는 항생제 치료가 필요하다.

④ 수술 전 항생제 사용에 대해서는 이식 팀과 상의한다.

⑤ 혈액배양 양성이나 확인된 감염이 장기 기증의 금기증은 아니다.

(13) 수혈 지침.

① Target Hemoglobin >7 g/dL, Hematocrit 21%이상

② Hb 7 g/dL 미만인 경우 충전 적혈구(PL-RBC)를 수혈한다.

③ Platelet, FFP 등은 혈액응고장애의 정도에 따라 수혈한다.

④ 수혈은 이식환자와 같이 filter된 혈액(PL-RBC, SDP or LD-PC) 으로 수혈한다.

(14) Lab follow up

① Initial 검사: General Examination

② Daily 정규 lab, chest X-ray

③ 선정장기에 따른 PRN 항목 추가

2. Deceased Donor Management Protocol

1) Check V/S q 1hr c continuous monitoring

2) BR

3) NPO

4) Check I/O q 8hrs c HUO

5) Check CVP monitoring q 8hr

6) ** Minimum target **

   MAP > 75 mmHg

   UO > 1 cc/kg/hr

   BT > 34℃ Na < 155 mEq

   P/F ratio > 200 (폐기증시 > 350)

7) Keep A-line with continuous monitoring

8) Check B. Wt & Ht.

9) Keep Foley cath.

10) L-tube natural drainage

11) Position change q 2hr

12) Ventilator care

   HOB 30도 이상

   Stress ulcer prophylaxis

13) PRN lab f/u q 6hrs

14) Continuous RI protocol

   Check BST q 6hrs

   Target BST 150 (140~180)

15) Vasopressors

   Vasopressin 0.03 IU/min (NE > 0.05 or Dopa >5인 경우 start)

   Norepinephrine ( ) mcg/kg/min (start from 0.05)

   Dopamine ( ) mcg/kg/min (start from 5)

   Dobutamine ( ) mcg/kg/min (start from 3)

16) Cortisolu 100 mg IV bolus & 200 mg CIV over 24hrs

17) 수술전 blood culture f/u. 수술 전 anti 확인.

18) 0.45% saline or 5% DW 40 cc/hr (상태에 따라 증감)

19) Famotidine 20 mg c x5dw50 IV bid

20) Cortisolu 100 mg IV loading

21) Cortisolu 200 mg c 5% DW 100 mL CIV over 24hrs

22) Prn) furosemide 10 mg IV for I/O control

23) 검사처방 ; 뇌사판정절차 참조.

CHAPTER 05.

LIVER TRANSPLANTATION RECIPIENT EVALUATION AND PREPARATION

I. Evaluation of Liver transplant recipient

1. Past medical history

  1) Cause of liver transplantation

  2) Liver Cirrhosis Complications

    (1) Varix: Endoscopic finding, EVL Hx, bleeding Hx

    (2) Ascites: Ascites control (Diuretics/Tapping), SBP

    (3) Hepatic Encephalopathy

  3) HBV-related: Anti-viral agent, YMDD mutation

  4) HCV-related: Anti-viral therapy, HCV Genotype

  5) HCC – previous treatment: TACE, RFA, Resection, Recent F/U

    - If the patient had Radiotherapy, considering Hepatico-jejuno than duct-to-duct anastomosis.

6) Co-morbid condition

: Hepato-Renal syndrome, Hepato-Pulmonary syndrome

2. Current status of the liver

1) Liver function test including coagulation profile and platelet count

2) Lipid profile

3) MELD score or PELD score

4) Hepatitis profile with HBV DNA quantitation, HCV RNA quantification

5) Doppler US, EGD

6) Liver CT: HCC, vasculature - R/O PV thrombosis

7) PET-CT: HCC patient

Liver MRI – SMC gadolinium protocol

3. Current infection

: chapter 3 ˈInfection in transplantation recipientsˈ 참조.

4. Malignancy

: Liver CT, Chest CT (metastasis protocol), Bone scan, PET-CT, Tumor marker (CEA, AFP, PIVKA-II, CA19-9), Mammography (F), Cervicovaginal smear (F)

(meta w/u: Chest CT/Bone scan q3Mo f/u)

5. Cardiovascular evaluation

1) ECG Routine, Advanced Echo

2) Carotid duplex scan : 60세 이상에서만 시행.

3) If PortoPulmonary HTN is suspected, consult cardiology.

6. HLA Test

1) Perform POD # -1, if there is no result.

   HLA-A,B typing (DNA), HLA-DR Typing (DNA),

   HLA crossmatch, HLA crossmatch (Flow cytometry)

   PRA screening, HLA class I, II

2) In case of ABOiLT, HLA test is performed before administra-tion of rituximab.

7. Consultation

: Infectious deparment, Dentistry, ENT, Psychiatry, NST, Rehabilitation, Social Welfare Office, Obstetrics and Gynecology (Women)

  Cardiology as needed.

8. West-Haven Criteria for Hepatic Encephalopathy (HE)

Stage	Consciousness	Intellect and Behavior	Neurologic Findings
0	Normal	Normal	Normal exam; if impaired psychomotor testing, consider MHE
1	Mild lack of awareness	Shortened attention span	Impaired addition or subtraction; mild asterixis or tremor

2	Lethargic	Disoriented; Inappropriate behavior	Obvious asterixis; Slurred speech
3	Somnolent but arousable	Gross disorientation; Bizarre behavior	Muscular rigidity and clonus; Hyperreflexia
4	Coma	Coma	Decerebrate posturing

9. Model for End-Stage Liver Disease: MELD Score

1) MELD Score: Three month-survival in waiting list

   MELD score= $9.57 \times \log_e$ Creatinine mg/dL

   $+ 3.78 \times \log_e$ Bilirubin mg/dL

   $+ 11.20 \times \log_e$ INR

   $+ 6.43$ (constant for liver disease etiology)

2) PELD Score

   PELD score= $0.436 \times$ (Age)

   $- 0.687 \times \log_e$ Albumin g/dL

   $+ 0.480 \times \log_e$ Bilirubin mg/dL

   $+ 1.857 \times \log_e$ INR

   $+ 0.667 \times$ (growth failure)

   (Age <1: score 1; Age > 1 : score 0

   Growth failure - 2 Standard deviations below mean for age : score 1 ≤ 2 SD below mean for age: score 0)

10. HCC in LT

1) Milan criteria (Mazzaferro et al, N Engl J Med, 1996;334:693)

   (1) Single HCC ≤ 5 cm in diameter

   (2) Multiple tumors ≤ 3 tumor nodules (each ≤ 3 cm in diameter)

2) UCSF criteria   (Yao et al, Hepatology 2001;33:1394)

  (1) Solitary tumor $\leq$ 6.5 cm

  (2) $\leq$ 3 nodules with the largest $\leq$ 4.5 cm

    (total tumor diameter $\leq$ 8 cm)

11. LT in Acute liver failure: King' s College Criteria

  1) Paracetamol (acetaminophen) overdose

    (1) $H^+>$50 nmol/L

      or all of the following:

    (2) Prothrombin time > 100 seconds

    (3) Creatinine > 300 umol/L

    (4) Grade III-IV encephalopathy

  2) Non-paracetamol (acetaminophen)

    (1) Prothrombin time > 100 seconds

      Or three of the following:

    (2) Age < 10 years or > 40 years

    (3) Prothrombin time > 50 seconds

    (4) Bilirubin > 300 μmol/L

    (5) Time from jaundice to encephalopathy > 2 days

    (6) Non-A, non-B hepatitis, halothane or drug-induced acute liver
      failure

12. 간장대기자 등록 서식

간장응급도 1 등록 서식

KONOS ID : 대기자명 :	(성인)	등록기관명: 책임자성명:　　　　　　(인)

정보

•성　명 : _____　•생년월일 : ___ 년 ___ 월 ___ 일　• 성별 : □ 남자　□ 여자

•등록일 : ___ 년 ___ 월 ___ 일　•관리일자 : ___ 년 ___ 월 ___ 일

임상 정보

•체중 : ___ kg •신장 : ___ cm •혈액형: □ A □ B □ O □ AB •Rh : □ + □ −

• 진단명 : □ 급성 간부전 □ 윌슨병 □ 기타(_____)

Serology	검사항목	양성	음성	검사항목	양성	음성
	HBs Ag			Anti-HCV		
	HBs Ab			Anti-HIV		
	Anti-HBc IgM			VDRL		

과거이식여부 : □ 아니오　□ 예　1차 장기명 _____　이식일자_____

2차 장기명 _____　이식일자_____

응급도 1 등록 기준

– 18세 이상의 전격성 간부전증(Fulminant liver failure)환자가 7일 이내에 간이식을 받지
않으면 생명 연장의 희망이 없는 상태로 다음 중 한가지 이상에 해당하는 경우

① 만성 간질환 없이 간질환의 증상이 나타난 후 8주 이내에 뚜렷한 간성혼수가 동반된 급성
전격성 간부전증(Fulminant liver failure)환자로, 중환자실에 입원 중이면서 다음의 3가지
조건중 한가지 이상을 동반한 경우

•인공호흡요법　• 신대체요법　• INR> 2.0

② 간이식후 7일 이내에 이식된 간이 기능을 하지 못하는 경우(Primary non-function)로 ㉮ 혹은
㉯ 조건을 동반한 경우 (단, 검사결과는 간이식 후 7일 이내 검사결과여야함.)
㉮ AST>=3,000이면서 다음의 2가지 조건중 하나 이상을 만족하는 경우
• INR>=2.5　•뚜렷한 산성혈증(acidosis, 동맥혈 PH<=7.30 혹은 정맥혈
PH<=7.25 이거나/혹은 Lactate>=4 mMol/L)
㉯ 무간상태(anhepatic state)

③ 윌슨병(Wilson's disease) 환자에게 급성 간부전증이 동반된 경우로 ① 항의 조건중 한가지
이상을 동반한 경우
① 항의 조건 : •인공호흡요법　• 신대체요법　• INR> 2.0

간장 이식대기자 응급도 등록관련 세부지침

응급등급 및 응급도	재등록 기간	검사결과 인정 범위		재등록 누락 시
응급등급 1	8일 이내 재등록	1회 연장, 총 14일 유지	서식지 통보	응급등급 2 이하의 으로 자동변환
응급등급 2, 3 (MELD 31-40)	8일 이내 재등록	(등록일 기준) 48시간 이내의 결과	등록 시 결과지 첨부	멜드점수 6점 자동변환, 수술 전 관리 1일 1회 제한, 재등록 기간은 마지막 재등록 시점 기준
응급등급 4 (MELD21-30)	3개월 이내 재등록	(등록일 기준) 14일 이내의 결과	이식자 선정 후 결과지 첨부	
응급등급 5 (MELD ≤ 20)	6개월 이내 재등록	(등록일 기준) 30일 이내의 결과		

II. Preparation of Adult Liver transplant recipient

1. Preparation for Transfusion:

전날 오후 3시 이전 처방이 들어가야 함.

1) Pre-storage leukocyte reduced RBC: 10U (irradiation and filtration)
2) FFP: 10 U
3) SDP 1U
4) Cryoprecipitate: 6U

2. To OR

1) Simulect 1V
2) Methylprednisolone 500 mg
3) Hepabig 10,000 U: HBV-related or Anti-HBc (+) Donor
   20,000 U: HBV DNA (+) or HBe Ag (+) Recipient

4) Antibiotics- Cefotaxime 2 g 2 vial, Ubacillin 1.5 g 4 vial

5) Alprostadil 20 mcg 5A (100 mcg, LDLT only)

6) Nafamostat 50 mg 1v (50 mg, LDLT only)

7) 5%Albumin 2 bottle (DDLT only)

3. Preparation of Intraop. Medication

* Medication

1) Nafamostat (1 vial=50 mg)
   • 300 mg mixed in 5DW 50 mL, 2cc/hr
2) Alprostadil (1 amp = 20 mcg)
   • 17.5 mcg/kg mixed in 5DW 50 mL, 4cc/hr
3) Dalteparin (1 vial = 10,000 IU/4mL)
   • 50 IU/kg mixed in NS 50cc. (If Bwt> 60 kg 1.2 mL), 2 cc/hr
   # Mix the above three drugs, fill in 50 cc bag, put the type and amount of medicine on the sticker. Mix the medicine and give it to anesthesia department. It was agreed to use an anesthetic syringe pump.
   * Administration is started immediately after reperfusion, aseptic preparation during the anhepatic phase is needed.

4. Others

1) HBV DNA and antiviral medication Hx prior to transplantation.
2) Malnutrition, old age before and after transplan-tation: rehabilitation, nutrition consultation
3) Hepabig Dosage
   10,000 U: HBV-related recipient, or Donor's Anti-HBc (+)

20,000 U: Recipient's HBV DNA (+) or HBeAg (+) case

4) Patients with several TACE and RFA history

1개월 내 CT or MRI에서 seeding이나 metastasis 소견 없어야 함.

CHAPTER 06

LIVING LIVER DONOR EVALUATION AND MANAGEMENT

I. Pretransplant evaluation:

1차로 CT volumetry 상에서 size가 합격이면 2차로 MRCP, fibroscan 피검사 진행.

원칙적으로 vascular, biliary anatomy에 따른 contraindication 없음.

1. Volumetry (Donor): CT angiography - Vascular anatomy and Liver volume

GRWR이 0.8 이상, remnant liver가 30% 이상인 경우에 진행. 하지만 donor와 recipient의 나이 및 physical status에 따라 약간씩 다름.

1) Standard liver volume (SLV) of recipient = 706.2 × (BSA) + 2.4 = cm³ (BSA (m²) = Weight (kg) × Height (cm)/3600)

2) GRWR: Graft to Recipient Body Weight Ratio (>0.8%)

3) GV/SLV: SLV에 대한 Graft Volume의 Ratio (>40%)

	Donor		Recipient	
	Volume	%	GRWR	GV/SLV
Whole liver	cm^3			
Right lobe (excluding MHV)	cm^3	%	%	%
Left lobe (including MHV)	cm^3	%	%	%

How to measure estimated Graft volume, manually.

- Portal inflow기준: Right PV과 left PV의 territory 의 경계면이 transection plan임. 대부분의 경우 이 plane에 middle hepatic vein이 위치하지만 예외적인 경우가 있으므로 portal vein의 주행방향을 우선 확인해야함.

- 대부분의 경우 Middle hepatic vein이 IVC로 들어가는 지점과 GB fossa를 연결하는 Cantlie's line이 transection plane이 됨. 하지만 Portal inflow나 hepatic venous outlow에 variation이 있는 경우에는 portal inflow의 territory를 정확히 구분해야 함

- 본원 CT 중 5 mm cut을 이용하여 Excel에서 계산함.

- 타원 CT로 몇 mm cut인지 모르는 경우. Coronal view에서 맨 위에서 맨 아래까지 길이(A)를 측정한 뒤, coronal reconstruction에 사용된 axial phase의 slice cut 개수(B)로 나누어주면(A/B) 몇 mm cut인지 알 수 있음.

2. Venous outflow territory volume measurement

1) Measurement performed by Department of Radiology

Graft 크기를 100%로 놓고 RHV, RIHV, V5, V8 hepatic vein의 volume %측정

2) Guidance for performing venous outflow reconstruction during LT

3) Volumetry와 Venous territory를 LDLT당일 OR에 부착하고 확인함.

4) V5/V8 reconstruction은 사전에 측정한 volume과 perfusion시 flow 를 확인 후 reconstruction여부 결정함.

3. Evaluation for Fatty change

1) fibroscan, MRCP로 w/u

2) IntraOp. Liver Biopsy (Frozen) : < 30% (Macrovesicular fatty change)

   (1) MRI, Proton density fat fraction (PDFF) on M DIXON image : Rt lobe에서 3~4개 정도 위치에서 ROI 측정 후 average로 결정: MRI 에서 15%이상으로 예측되는 경우, preoperative biopsy 고려

   (2) Evaluation of Fatty change with CT scan: Pre-enhance scan with oval ROI (Region of Interest): CTL-S (difference liver-spleen attenuation): < -9 (or −7)이면 Bx. Recommended

4. Other preoperative work-up

1) Routine Lab

   (1) CBC with diff., Chemistry, electrolyte, TG, HDL-C, LDL-C, ABO/Rh typing & Ab screen (T&S), UA c micro., Stool Exam

   (2) PT/aPTT, Protein C activity

   (3) Chest PA, EKG, PFT

   (4) CT angiography

   (5) MRCP

(6) Liver fibroscan

(7) 2D echo: 65세 이상인 경우 해당

2) Evaluation for infectious disease

Serologic tests: HBsAg, anti-HBs Ab, anti-HBc Ab (IgG), anti-HCV Ab, anti-HAV Ab (IgG), Anti-HIV combo, RPR, TB Specific Interferone-Gamma (QTF), CMV Ab (IgG), EB-VCA (IgG), VZV Ab (IgG), Toxoplasma Ab (IgG), HSV Type 1 & 2 Ab (IgG)

3) 결과에 따른 기증자 전처치

(1) Stool exam 결과에서 Clonorchis Sinensis 소견이 보이면 praziquantel을 처방한다. 용량 25 mg/kg / 1회 * 하루 3회

(2) Anti-HBs Ab 음성이면 vaccination (Hepatitis B 1 mL, IM) 1회 시행 이후 1달 뒤 Anti-HBs Ab f/u하여 항체 생성여부를 확인하여 2,3차 접종 필요성을 평가 (감염내과 외래 진료 의뢰)

(3) Anti-HAV Ab (IgG) 음성이면 vaccination (Hepatitis A 1mL, IM) 시행. 6~12개월 뒤 2차 접종위해 감염내과 외래 진료 의뢰

(4) QTF 양성이면 non-contrast Chest CT 시행, QTF indeterminate이면 TB Specific Interferone-Gamma (T-SPOT)으로 재검 후 감염내과 외래 진료 의뢰

5. Consultation to other departments

1) Psychiatric: 『장기 등 기증자 및 장기 등 이식대기자의 신체검사 항목』중 살아있는 사람으로서 장기등 기증시 정신건강의학과 진료항목 신설.

2) Hepatology: 필요 시

3) Infection: (Other preoperative work up-결과에 따른 기증자 전처치)에 기술되어 있는 경우 협진 의뢰

4) Gynecology: 여성인 경우

5) Social service team: 상담평가를 위한 협진

6. 기증자 지문등록

장기 등 이식에 관한 법률 제 19조에 따라 상담 평가 및 본인여부 확인을 위해 시행 장기이식센터, 사회사업팀, 수술장에서 확인

7. 승인: 국립장기이식관리센터(KONOS)로부터 수술 전 승인을 받는다.

II. Follow up after discharge

1) First follow-up: 퇴원 후 2주 뒤, 기본 lab
2) Second follow-up: 4주 뒤에 CT follow up
3) From third follow-up: 3개월 뒤 Hepatology donor clinic시작

CHAPTER 07.

LIVER TRANSPLANTATION PROCEDURES

I. Deceased donor organ harvest (Liver)

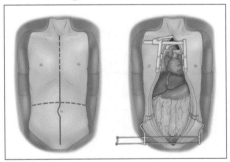

- Skin drape는 최대한 넓은 범위를 닦는다. Thoracotomy를 하는 경우 chin 이하 neck, shoulder까지 닦으며 suprapublic area까지 닦는다.
- Abdominal incision만 넣는 경우 long midline(빨간 실선) incision 을 사용하며, thoracotomy를 하는 경우 midline incision을 흉부까지 extension(빨간 점선)한다. 더 나은 exposure를 위해서 supraumbilical level에서 bilateral transverse incision을 넣을 수도 있다.
- Sternotomy와 long midline incision에 쓸 retractor를 apply하며, 양쪽 rib cage를 retract하기 위해 Iron Intern이나 Kent, Omni retractor 등을 사용한다.

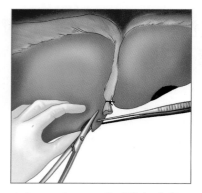

- Abdominal cavity에 진입한 뒤에는 liver biopsy를 시행한다. Liver 의 texture, elasticity, color, size 등을 평가하여 frozen biopsy상에서 steatosis, fibrosis, inflammation 소견 등과 종합하여 harvest를 진행할 지 결정한다.

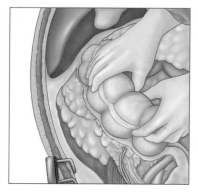

- Right side colon mobilization을 시행한다(Cattell-Braasch maneuver). 이를 통해 Right kidney, IVC, aorta를 expose한다. 이때, right ureter에 injury를 입히지 않도록 plane을 잘 들어가야 하며 colon과 duodenum을 함께 mobilization하면서 perirenal fat과 ureter는 하부에 남도록 한다.

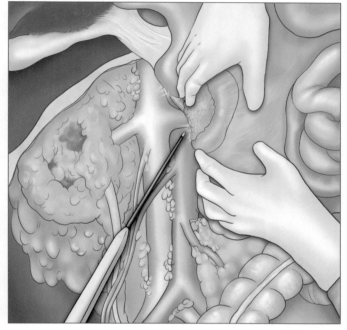

- Duodenum과 pancreas head도 mobilization한다. 윗쪽으로는 IVC와 left renal vein까지 expose하며 SMA 기시부 또한 나오게끔 한다. 아래쪽 에서는 aorta의 iliac bifurcation까지 expose하며 IMA 기시부도 나오게 끔 한다.

- Mobilization과정에서는 peritoneum을 bovie로 연 다음에는 손가 락을 이용한 blunt dissection하는 것이 정확한 plane을 따라 빠르게 dissection하는데 도움을 준다.

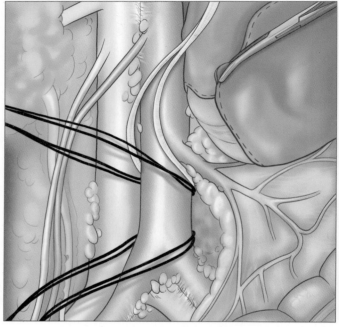

- Aorta isolation을 하기 위해 small bowel과 right colon을 큰 pad로 감싼 후 왼쪽 위로 당겨서 고정해둔다. IMA와 iliac bifurcation 사이의 aorta 사이에 1-0 silk tie 두 개를 위아래로 걸어두고 윗쪽으로는 nylon tape를 걸어둔다. 그 사이에 vertebral artery가 두 개 있을 수 있기 때문에 ligation하여 backflow가 발생하는 것을 예방한다. IMA level까지 aorta를 손가락으로 잡을 수 있을 정도로 mobilization해둔다.

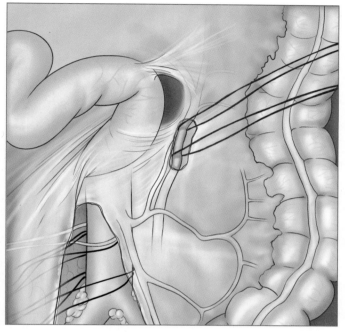

- IMV isolation을 위해 ligament of Treitz 옆으로 지나가는 부위에서 위 아래로 silk tie를 걸어둔다. Pancreas 구득을 하는 경우에는 catheter tip이 너무 올라가지 않도록 낮은 위치에서 확보한다.
- Left kidney의 cooling을 위하여 left colon mobilization을 시행하여 perirenal fat이 expose 될 수 있도록 한다.

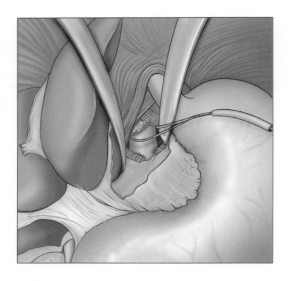

- Supraceliac aorta를 isolation하기 위해 liver left lateral lobe를 mobilization한다.

- Lesser omentum을 open한다. 이때, left gastric artery에서 liver로 들어 가는 aberrant left hepatic artery가 있는 경우 ligation하면 안된다.

- Liver left lobe와 caudate lobe를 같이 retraction한 상태에서 손가락으로 aorta의 pulsation을 느낀 뒤 visceral peritoneum과 그 안의 muscle layer를 bovie로 열면서 aorta를 expose한다.

- Aorta를 싸고 있는 connective tissue를 최대한 연 뒤에, long right angle로 aorta의 후면을 돌리고(오른손을 이용해서 aorta의 왼쪽으로 진 입하고 오른쪽으로 빼면서 술자의 왼손가락으로 tip을 촉지한다) nylon tape을 걸어 두고 tourniquet을 끼워둔다. 이 술식을 할 때, aorta에서 나 오는 작은 branch에 injury주지 않도록 right angle의 tip이 transverse하 게 돌릴 수 있도록 한다.

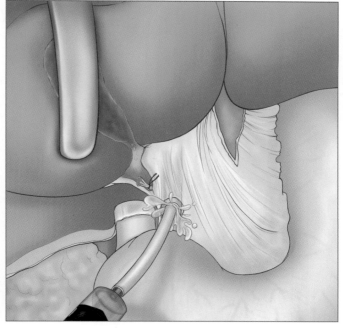

- Cholecystectomy하기 전에 hepatic artery의 pulsation을 촉지한다. SMA 에서 올라오는 right hepatic artery가 있는 경우 portal vein의 우측으로 가는 게 느껴진다.

- Cholecystectomy를 한 뒤에, hepatoduodenal ligament를 연 뒤, CBD하 부를 isolation한다. duodenum쪽으로 바짝 붙여서 tie ligation하고 그 위 의 CBD를 열고 normal saline으로 irrigation한다. 나오는 bile이 거의 없 어질 때까지 50 cc syringe를 이용해 여러 번 irrigation한다.

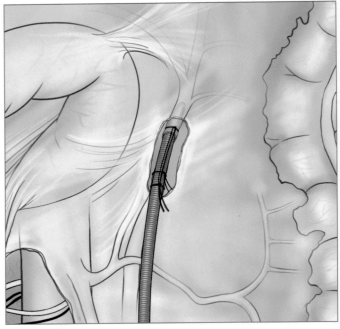

- Cannulation하기 전에 systemic heparin을 준다(한국 평균 성인 기준 25,000 U 정도).

- IMV cannulation을 시행한다. 미리 isolation해둔 IMV의 distal part을 tie 한 뒤 cut down method로 catheterization한다. Proximal end가 너무 깊이 들어가지 않도록 한다. Proximal tie를 이용하여 catheter를 tagging 하고 distal tie를 이용하여 재차 고정해준다.

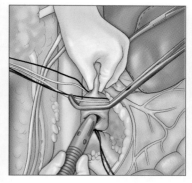 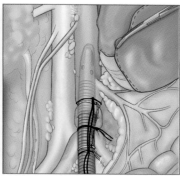

- Aorta cannulation을 위해 proximal clamping을 위한 적당한 size의 Satinsky clamp를 준비한다.

- Distal aorta를 tie한다. 이후에 proximal part에 Satinsky clamp를 이용해 clamping을 시행한다. 그리고 Metzenbaum scissor로 aortotomy incision을 넣는다.

- Surgeon은 왼손으로 clamping된 aorta의 proximal part을 손으로 막고, assistant는 Satinsky clamp를 declamping할 준비를 한다. Scrub nurse는 cannulation catheter의 rubber connector에 clamping되어 있는 clamp를 declamp-reclamp할 준비를 한다. Circulating nurse는 HTK perfusion 준비를 하고 얼음이 준비되어 있는지 확인한다.

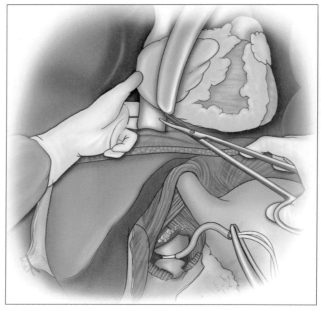

- Supraceliac aorta를 tourniquet을 이용하여 clamping을 시행하고 곧 바로 aorta와 IMV에 연결되어 있는 HTK solution을 declamping하여 perfusion을 시행한다.

- 미리 expose시켜둔 suprahepatic IVC를 opening한다. 자르는 위치는 심장 적출이 없는 경우 최대한 심장에 붙여서 자르며, 심장적출이 있는 경우 해당 의료진과 상의 하에 결정한다.

- IVC를 opening함과 동시에 Suction cap을 씌운 suction을 이용해 venous blood를 suction하여 뜨거운 피가 고이지 않도록 한다. 미리 준비된 얼음을 retrohepatic, subhepatic, 양쪽 kidney 위, 그리고 liver 위에 넣은 뒤, liver와 kidney의 색을 보면서 perfusion이 잘 진행되는지 확인한다.

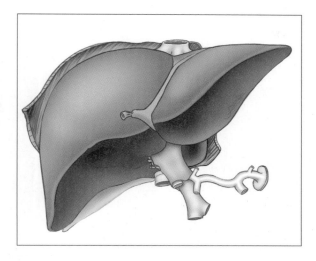

Cold dissection

① CBD transection

② RGA, GDA찾고 자르기→ GDA에서 CHA를 따라간뒤→Splenic artery까
지 찾고 적당한 stump를 두고 자르기→Celiac artery를 따라가면서 LGA
자르고→Aorta까지 접근한 후, celiac artery와 aorta 사이의 tissue를 자
른다. →Aorta를 expose한 뒤 celiac artery는 aorta patch 형태로 잘라
온다.

③ Portal vein은 SMV와 Splenic vein이 만나는 부위에서 각각 잘라온다.

④ Left renal vein과 right renal vein이 IVC와 합쳐지는 부위 상방의 IVC
를 자른다.

⑤ Right kidney를 아래로 내리면서 right adrenal gland를 절개하면서 liver
를 뗀다.

⑥ suprahepatic IVC opening에 손가락을 걸고 IVC와 liver의 injury를 방지
하면서 diaphragmatic muscle들을 자른다.

II. Laparoscopic Living Donor Hepatectomy

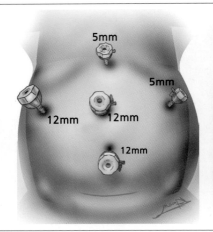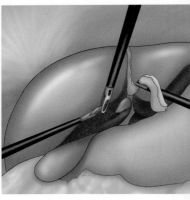

- Port insertion: 기본적으로 scope포함 다섯 개.
- Periumbilical port는 scope용으로 사용하며 일반적으로 배꼽의 하방에 삽입하지만 환자 체형에 따라, 배꼽, 또는 배꼽 위에 설치하기도 함.
- 나머지 port는 뱃속에서 간의 위치를 보고 조금씩 조정하여 설치한다.
- Liver biopsy (frozen)를 시행한다.

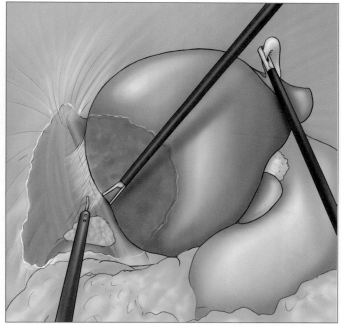

- Right liver mobilization: Right triangular ligament부터 시작해서 IVC 까지 medial side로 full mobilization시행한다.

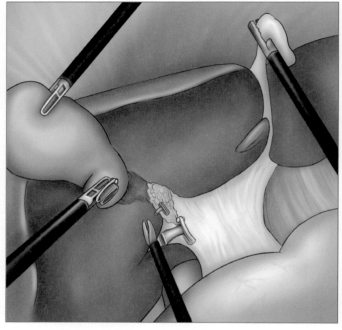

- Partial cholecystectomy: Cystic duct stump가 최대한 길게 남도록 cholecystectomy를 시행하되 GB를 GB bed에서 완전히 떼지 않고 retraction 목적으로 남겨둔다.

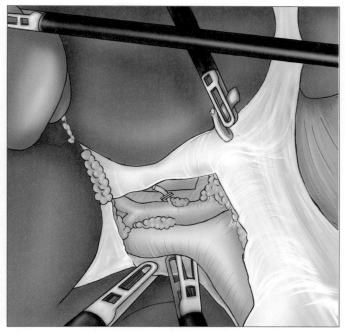

- 보조의가 GB와 cystic duct stump를 잡고 hilum을 보여주면 hepatoduodenal ligament를 절개하여 내부로 접근하여 right hepatic artery와 right portal vein을 dissection한다.

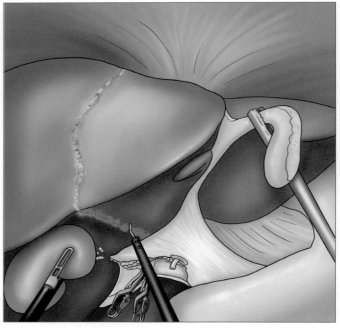

- Bulldog clamp를 이용하여 right hepatic artery와 right portal vein
을 temporary clamping하고 Cantlie's line에 생기는 demarcation
을 bovie로 marking한다. Liver의 inferior surface쪽에는 bile duct
bifurcation 부위까지 이은 선에 marking한다.

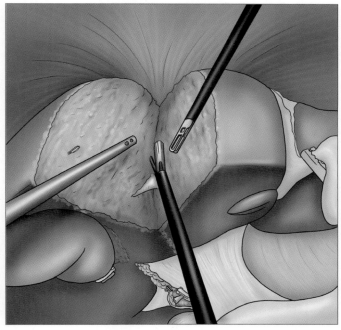

- Bulldog clamp를 제거한 뒤 parenchymal transection을 시작한다. 보
조의는 왼손으로는 ligamentum teres를 이용하고 오른손으로는 grasper
로 traction한다. 집도의는 gallbladder와 suction 등을 이용하여 traction
한다.

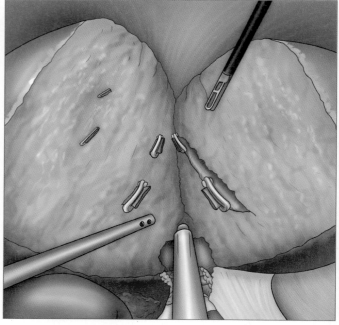

- Middle hepatic vein은 left side (remnant liver)에 붙인 채로 transection을 진행하고 V5/V8 branch들은 hem-o-lok polymer clip을 이용하여 ligation한다.

- Bile duct가 expose되는 부위에서부터는 thermal damage를 줄이기 위해 CUSA를 이용한다.

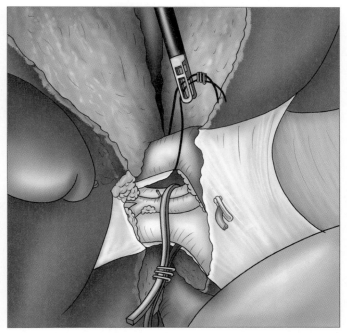

- Right portal vein과 right hepatic artery를 완전히 isolation한 뒤, vessel loop으로 걸어둔다.

- 보조의가 vessel loop이나 cystic duct등을 retraction하여 caudate가 expose되게 하면 caudate lobe도 transection하여 bile duct posterior side를 encircling 가능하게끔 한다. 이후 Right-angle을 이용하여 silk를 통과시킨 뒤 bile duct만 isolation한다.

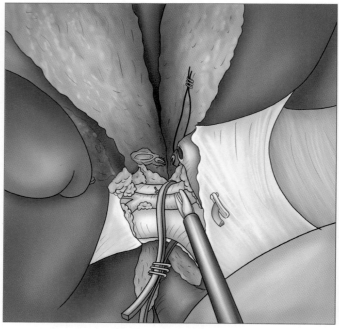

- 보조의가 silk를 살짝 당긴 상태에서 CHD와 RHD의 conjunction을 identification한 뒤 scissor를 이용하여 bile duct를 절개한다. 이후 duct posterior side로 있는 Glisson tissue는 clipping한다.

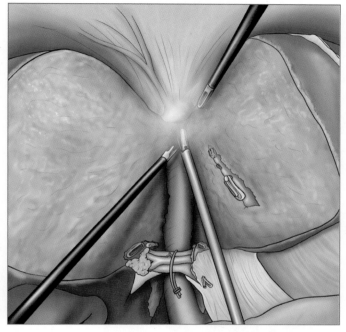

- IVC와 caudate lobe 사이를 dissection하면서 나머지 부위 transection
  을 시행한다.

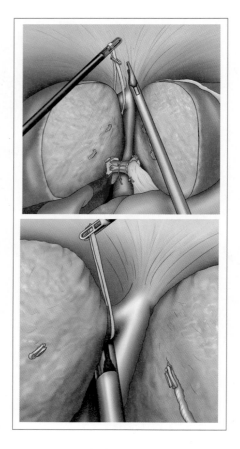

- RHV를 isolation한 뒤 nylon tape로 걸어둔다.
- IVC에 붙어있는 부위를 마저 detach시켜주고 IVC ligament가 있는 부위는 laparocopic GIA stapler로 ligation한다.

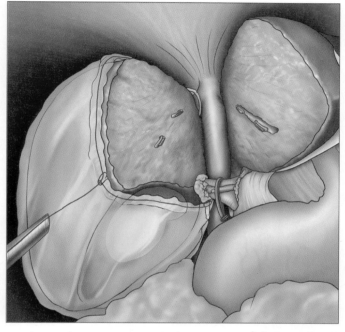

- Portal vein, hepatic artery, right hepatic vein 외의 구조물이 모두 detach된 이후에 laparoscopic plastic bag에 넣은 뒤 GB를 마저 떼어 넣어둔다.

- 이후에 Pfannenstiel incision을 통해 laparoscopic bag의 끈을 빼두고 temporary closure 시행해둔다.

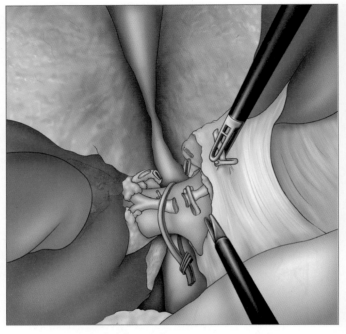

- Heparin 5,000 IU을 마취과를 통해 IV administration한다
- Right hepatic artery를 hem-o-lok clip으로 잡고 distal은 scissor로 자른다.

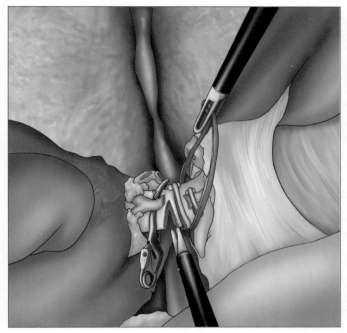

- 보조의가 vessel loop을 살짝 left side로 잡은 채로 큰 hem-o-lok으로
  Portal vein을 clipping한다. 이때, portal vein stricture가 생기지 않도록
  주의한다.
- Distal right portal vein은 bulldog clamp로 잡아두고 portal vein은
  clip에서 1 mm이상의 stump를 둔 채로 자른다.

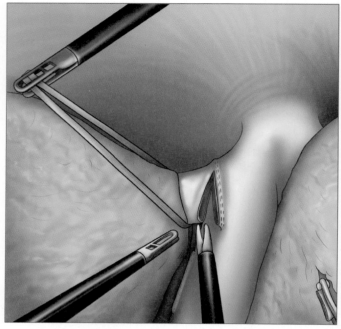

- 보조의가 RHV에 걸려있는 nylon tape를 right anterior side로 full traction을 한 상태에서 laparoscopic TA stapler를 이용해 IVC side로 최대한 붙여서 stapling한다.
- Scissor를 이용해서 RHV를 자른다.
- 이후 liver graft는 bag안에 담은 뒤 Pfannenstiel incision을 통해 rapid deliver로 한다.

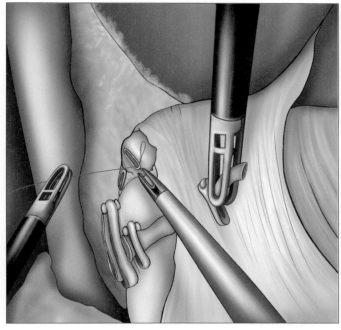

- Bleeding control을 시행 한 뒤, remnant bile duct opening은 ligation 하도록 한다.
- Falciform ligament는 다시 suture로 고정해둔다.

III. Backtable Procedures

1. Perfusion with preservation solution

2. Graft delivery 후에 graft에 연결되어 있는 bulldog clamp 등을 제거 후에 pre-perfusion weight를 측정한다.

3. Portal vein에 HTK solution catheter를 위치시킨 뒤 assistant가 붙잡고 있도록 한다. 한 손으로 catheter를 잡고 나머지 손은 forcep으로 portal vein의 입구로 잡아서 조여주도록 한다.

4. Perfusion 시작 후에 major hepatic vein으로 flushing이 되는 것을 확인하도록 한다. Catheter의 위치와 방향에 따라 preservation solution이 들어가지 않을 수 있으므로 지속적으로 HTK solution bag에서 용액이 잘 내려가는지 확인한다.

5. V5와 V8의 hem-o-lok을 제거하기 전에 liver의 anterior surface에 right anterior section의 congestion 범위가 어느 정도 되는지 눈으로 확인한다.

6. V5와 V8의 hem-o-lok을 제거한 뒤에는 hepatic artery에 flushing시작한다.

7. Main portal vein의 길이가 짧은 경우에는 HTK solution이 right anterior 나 right posterior 중 한 방향으로 많이 흘러 들어갈 수 있으므로 flushing되는 용액에 혈액이 얼마만큼 나오는지 보고 개별적으로 flushing 해보기도 한다.

8. Perfusion이 종료된 이후에 post-perfusion weight를 측정한다.

9. Benchwork

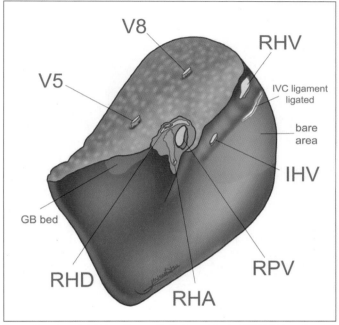

Figure. Overview of right hemiliver graft. Right portal vein RPV, Right hepatic artery RHA, Right hepatic duct RHD, Gallbladder GB, Right hepatic vein RHV, Inferior vena cava IVC, Inferior hepatic vein IHV

- Benchwork의 첫 번째 목표는 graft가 recipient 몸속에 있는 warm ischemic time (hepatic vein anastomosis to reperfusion)을 최소화시키는 데 있음. 두 번째 목표는 graft entry부터 skin closure까지 최소의 시간이 소요되게끔 사전 준비하는 것임.

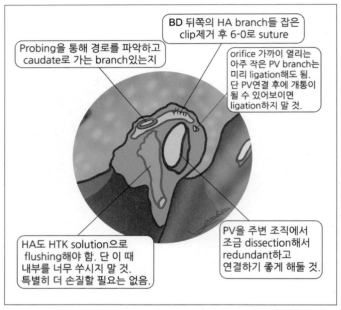

Figure. Backtable procedures for hilar region.

- Portal vein을 연결하기 좋게끔 길게 뽑아준다. Bile duct opening 후방
  에는 hepatic artery의 caudate branch가 있는데 clipping되어 있는 부
  분은 수술 중 suture가 걸리거나 빠질 수 있으므로 제거하고 다시 suture
  ligation해준다.

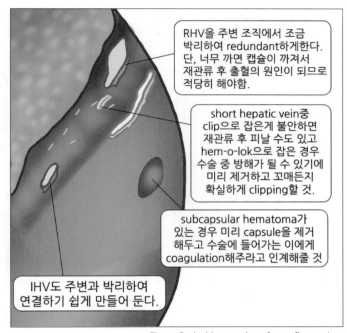

Figure. Backtable procedures for outflow regions

- Hepatic vein을 연결하기 좋게끔 길게 뽑아준다. Liver 뒤쪽의 clip을 모두 제거해줄 필요는 없으나 수술 중 탈락될 가능성이 커보이거나 hepatic vein opening 주변에 위치하여 suture 중에 걸릴 가능성이 높아보이는 경우 제거 후 suture ligation 하는 것을 고려해본다.

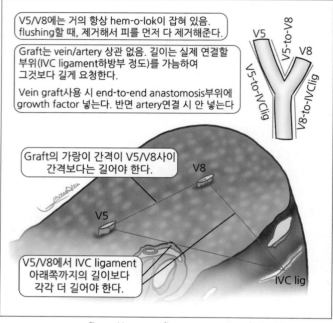

Figure. Venous outflow reconstruction of V5/V8 hepatic veins

- Outflow reconstruction에는 cryopreserved iliac vein graft가 선호되지만 Y-shape graft가 없는 경우 cryopreserved iliac artery graft를 사용한다.

- 그림과 같이 길이를 예상하여 graft를 준비하며 최소한 IVC ligament의 inferior half에 닿는 길이는 되어야 하지만 그 길이보다 여유있게 준비하는 것이 좋음.

- Vein을 쓰는 경우 내부에 valve가 있는지 확인하고 있는 경우 겉과 속을 뒤집어서 valve를 제거해준다. Artery를 쓰는 경우 내부에 atheroma가 있는지 확인하고 심하지 않은 경우 그대로 쓰지만 anastomosis 부위에

크게 있는 경우 intima가 damage입지 않게 조심스럽게 plaque를 제거
한다.

- 최종적으로 IVC에 연결할 것으로 예상되는 위치와 방향에 맞춰서 design
한다. Graft의 bifurcation위치는 예상 연결 부위보다 길어서는 안 된다.
- V5/V8 opening의 네군데 corner에 tagging suture를 넣어서 방향이 돌지
않도록 한다.
- Vein을 연결할 때, growth factor를 만들어준다. Artery를 쓸때는 만들지
않는다. Vein을 써도 IVC에 end-to-side로 연결하는 경우 growth factor
를 넣지 않는다.
- Prolene 6-0로 suture를 마친 뒤에 leakage test를 시행한다.

10. Preparation for cryopreserved vessels.

11. 인체조직포장 개봉방법

    2인 1조로 봉투를 개봉한다. 조직은 3중 포장되어 있음.

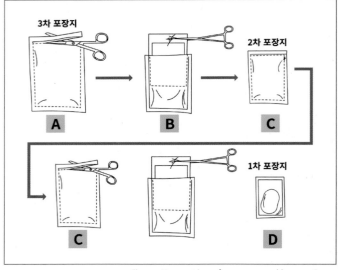

Figure. Unwrapping of cryopreserved human tissue.

1. 순회 간호사는 비닐봉지를 똑바로 세운 상태에서 가장 윗부분의 접합 부위를 알코솜을 이용하여 2~3회 문지른다. 이후 소독 간호사는 멸균 Mayo scissor를 이용하여 바깥쪽 비닐봉투를 자르고 Mayo scissor를 순회 간호사에게 전달한다. 이때 2차 비닐봉투가 손상되지 않도록 주의한다.

2. 순회 간호사가 3차 비닐봉투의 양쪽 모서리를 잡고 소독간호사는 무균 Kelly를 사하여 2차 비닐포장을 꺼낸다.

3. 소독간호사는 2차 비닐포장을 멸균 테이블에 놓고 멸균 Mayo scissor를 사용하여 2차 비닐봉투에 가장 윗부분을 잘라 1차 포장지를 꺼낸다.

4. 1차 비닐봉투를 42℃ 0.9% Normal Saline이 담긴 Bowl에 넣고 녹인다. 해동 과정은 42℃ 상태를 유지하면서 10분 이내에 실행한다.

12. 인체조직 해동 및 세척 과정

　1) 기구

　　(1) Bowl 3 ea

　　(2) Mayo scissor 3 ea

　　(3) Debakey forcep 1 ea

　　(4) Kelly or sponge forcep 2 ea

　　(5) Alcohol 솜

　　(6) Culture Bottle 1ea

　　(7) 37~42℃ 멸균 생리식염수

13. 해동과정(2인 1조)

　1) 인체조직은 3중 포장되어 있다. "인체조직 포장 개봉방법"에 따라 무균적으로 1차 비닐포장을 꺼낸다

　2) 포장 개봉 방법을 통해 꺼내진 1차 비닐포장을 37~42℃의 멸균생리식염수 Bowl에 넣는다.

　3) Bowl에 따뜻한 식염수를 첨가해서 42℃가 유지되도록 계속해서 따뜻한 식염수를 첨가한다. 얼음이 모두 녹을 때까지 적어도 5-10분간 담가서 녹인다. 42℃가 유지되도록 계속해서 따뜻한 식염수를 첨가한다. 얼음이 다 녹은 것을 확인하면 비닐 봉투를 부드럽게 흔들어 준다. 봉투는 계속 식염수 속에 있어야 한다. 얼음이 다 녹지 않았다고 손으로 짜면 얼음이 이식조직에 손상을 주므로 하지 말아야 한다.

　4) 해동이 완전히 끝나면 세척을 시작한다. 해동 후에 DMSO에 노출되는 시간이 길면 세포에 독성이 가해지므로 신속하게 세척을 한다.

14. 세척과정(단계적 세척)

　1) 해동된 1차 포장지를 멸균Scissor로 열고, Debakey Forcep 등을 사용해서 주의깊게 인체조직을 꺼낸다.

　2) 꺼내진 인체조직은 멸균 생리식염수가 담긴 각각의 Bowel에서 3분씩

2번 Passively 세척한다. 미리 2개의 Bowel에 37~42℃의 300~500 mL 의 멸균 생리식염수를 담아 놓는다.

3) 2번의 Rinsing 과정이 끝나면 인체조직은 사용 가능 상태가 된다. 사용 하기 전까지 멸균 생리식염수나 HTK 용액에 담아 놓는다. 이때 절대로 조직은 건조하게 만들면 안 된다.

IV. Recipient hepatectomy

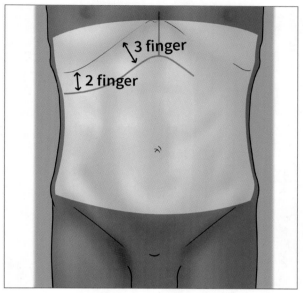

- Preparation: Draping후 sterile film (IobanTM)으로 cover한다. Surgical field 상방과 하방에 각각 일반 suction과 Cell saver용 suction을 각각 설치한다.

- Incision: Mercedez-Benz incision. Right subcostal incision은 medial side에서는 rib에서 3 finger, leteral side에서는 2 finger로 넣는다. Left subcostal incision은 right side에 대칭이 되도록 한다.

- 복강 내에 진입 후 복수를 일반 suction을 이용해서 suction 하도록 양을 count한다.

- Ligamentum teres와 falciform ligament를 ligation후 Iron-intern retaractor를 apply한다.

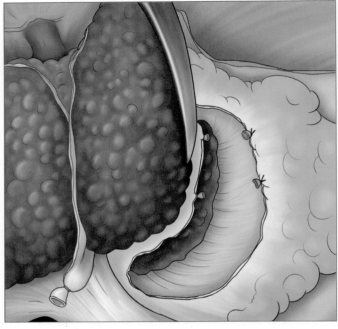

- Left triangulat ligament를 dissection한 뒤, left liver를 right side로 traction하고 lesser omentum부터 open한다. Hepatoduodenal ligament 옆의 투명한 부분부터 open한 뒤, 상방으로 진행한다. 중간에 vessel이 나오면 ligation하고, accessory or replaced left hepatic artery가 left gastric artery에서 나오는 경우, 결찰하지 않고 isolation만 해둔다.

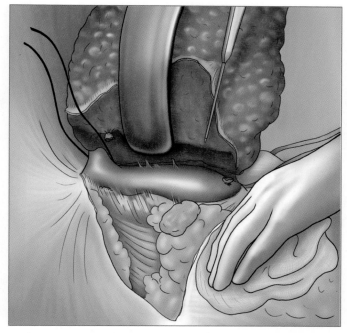

- Right liver도 mobilzation하고 caudate process와 IVC 사이의 plane으로 dissection한다. 하방에서 상방으로 올라가면서 short hepatic vein을 ligation한다. IVC ligament는 Satinsky로 잡고 suture ligation한다. Right hepatic vein을 silk tie로 걸어둔다.

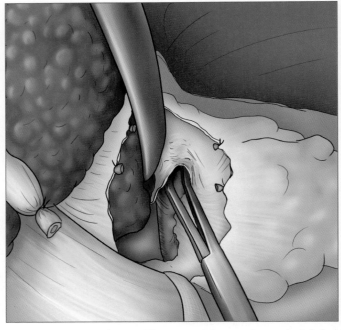

- IVC 반대편까지 dissection이 되면 left side에서 Spiegel's lobe와 복벽에 연결된 peritoneum을 open해주면서 left hepatic vein 위치까지 올라간다.

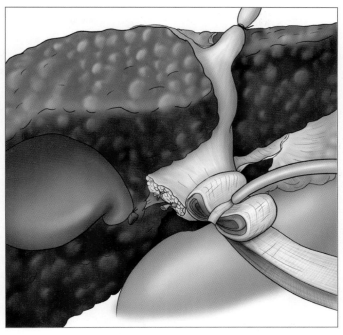

- Partial cholecystectomy 후 inflow control를 하여 anhepatic phase로 들어간다.
- 미리 걸어둔 right hepatic vein을 Satinsky clamp로 잡은 뒤 clamp-to-clamp로 고정한다. 이때 IVC를 지나치게 많이 잡을 경우 central venous return에 장애가 올 수 있으므로 주의한다.

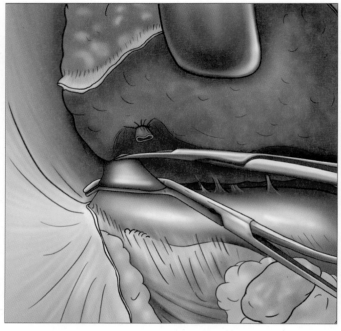

- Right hepatic vein을 liver parenchyme에 최대한 붙여서 길게 stump가 남도록 자른다.

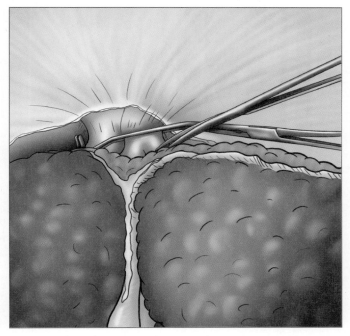

- Left hepatic vein과 middle hepatic vein의 common trunk를 Satinsky clamp로 잡은 뒤 마찬가지로 liver parenchyme에 최대한 붙여서 자른다.

- Right hepatic vein stump는 anatomosis에 이용할 것이므로 그대로 두고 left and middle hepatic vein stump를 Prolene 4-0 로 suture closure하도록 한다.

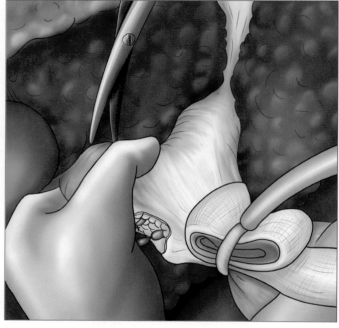

- Hilum을 자르기 전에 finger dissection을 통해 특히 right과 left가 갈라
  지는 hilar Glisson pedicle과 liver parenchyme 사이의 공간을 확보한
  뒤 Glisson pedicle을 길게 남도록 잘라준다.

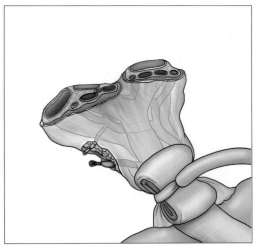

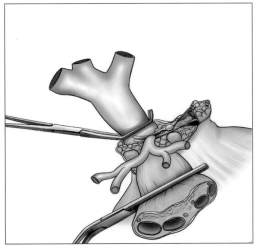

- Hilar dissection은 portal vein을 전방의 bile duct와 hepatic artery로
  부터 떼어내는 것부터 시작한다. Nylon tape이 걸려있는 level까지 내려

온 뒤, Satinsky와 iliac clamp 등을 이용해서 bleeding이 없도록 portal vein과 artery/duct를 각각 잡아두고 nylon tape는 푼다.

- Pancreas로 들어가는 level까지 portal vein을 dissection해서 redundant 하게 만들어준다.

- Inflow를 풀었다 잡았다 하면서 artery를 identification하고 artery를 bile duct에서 dissection해주고 proximal level에서 bulldog clamp로 잡아둔다. 이때 bile duct에 손상이 가지 않도록 주의한다. Bile duct는 iliac clamp로 잡아둔다.

- Hilar structure들은 차례대로 거즈와 포개어둔 뒤, iron intern retractor 의 아랫쪽 발을 이용하여 아래로 제쳐둔다.

- Recipient의 collateral circulation 여부에 따라 anhepatic phase의 시점을 조절할 수 있음. Collateral이 풍부한 경우, inflow control을 앞당겨서 hepatectomy를 시행하면 출혈과 시간을 단축할 수 있으므로 개별 환자의 상태에 맞춰서 진행할 수 있음.

- 하지만 collateral이 없는 상태에서 inflow를 차단 후 수술을 진행하면 이후에 inflow를 재개하는 경우 더 심한 출혈이 발생할 수 있으므로 donor 로부터 graft가 나오는 시점과 recipient hepatectomy가 종료될 시점을 맞추는 것이 바람직함.

V. Transplantation

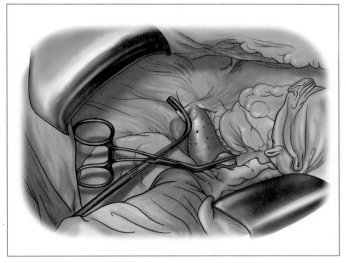

- Anhepatic phase에서 anastomosis가 잘될 수 있게끔, IVC도 적절하게 mobilization 해두고 portal vein도 주변 조직에서 detach시켜서 mobile 하게 만든다.

- Graft anastomosis 이후에는 수술 field가 좁아지므로 IVC 주변과 diaphragm, adrenal, perirenal fat 등에서 bleeding focus를 미리 지혈 (필요하면 suture ligation)하도록 한다.

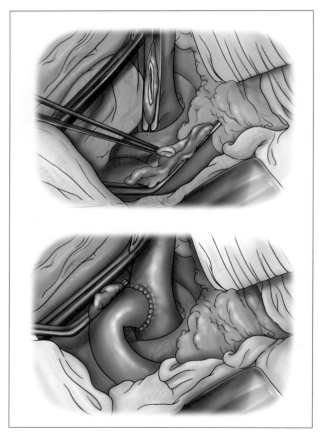

- Mesenteric blood flow가 차단된 상태에서 systemic circulation으로 우회하는 collateral vessel이 충분치 않은 경우 bowel congestion 및 hypovolemia가 올 수 있다. 이런 경우 left portal vein과 IVC를 임시로 연결해두는 portocaval shunt를 temporary하게 시행할 수 있음.

- Portocaval shunt는 reperfusion 후에 다시 closure시행할 수 있음.

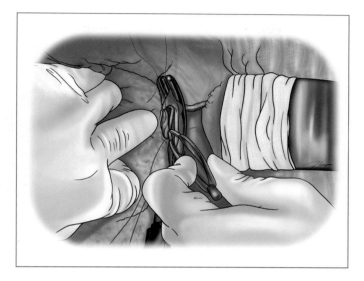

- 미리 측정한 graft RHV opening의 길이만큼 recipient RHV에 opening 을 만들어서 4-0 Prolene running suture로 anastomosis 시행한다. 양쪽 edge에 tagging suture를 한 뒤에 아랫쪽 tagging suture는 rubber shot mosquito로 잡고 아래로 당겨서 팽팽하게 만든다. 윗쪽 tagging suture를 세 차례 tie를 양쪽 길이가 같게 시행한 뒤 긴 실을 이용해서 혈관 안쪽으로 통과시킨 뒤 running suture를 시작한다.

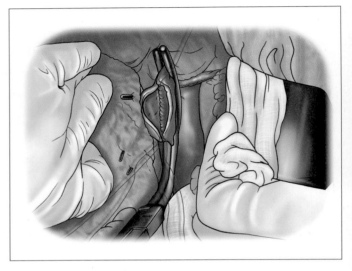

- Dorsal side부터 running suture로 내려온 후 아랫쪽 끝에서 바깥으로 실을 통과시킨다. 미리 tagging suture해둔 아랫쪽 실을 세 차례 tie한 뒤, 짧은 실과 running suture로 내려온 실을 여섯 번 tie한다. Tie를 시행한 두 실은 rubber shot mosquito로 잡아둔 뒤 팽팽하게 당겨둔다.

- 나머지 긴 실을 이용하여 ventral side의 혈관 벽을 running suture로 시행한다. Backward suture로 서너 땀 뜨면서 올라간 뒤, 윗쪽에서 남은 실을 가지고 내려온다.

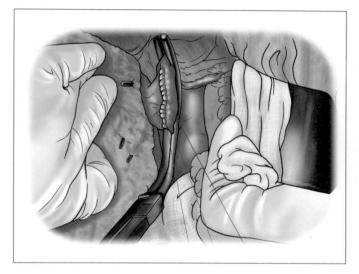

- 위아래에서 가운데로 모인 running suture는 가운데에서 6번 tie한다.
  Growth factor를 주지 않는다.

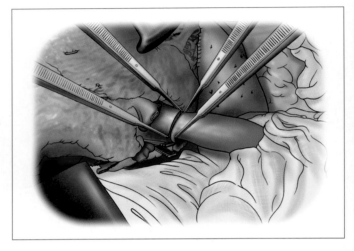

- Portal vein anastomosis를 위해서 recipient portal vein의 길이를 측정하고 적절한 위치에서 남는 vein을 자른다. 지나친 tension은 stircture를 유발할 수 있고 지나치게 redundant한 경우 natural flow에 장애가 발생할 수 있다.

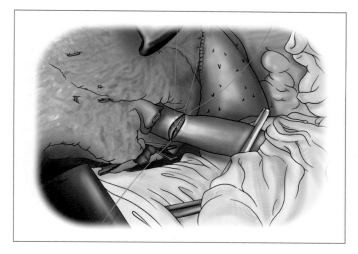

- Vein의 축이 돌지 않도록 정확한 위치에 tagging suture를 시행하고 3차
  례씩 tie를 시행한다. 윗쪽 실부터 내부로 통과하여 running suture를 시
  행한다. 이때, 지나치게 실을 당기지 않는 것이 중요하며 approximation
  되는 정도의 tension으로 실을 잡아준다.

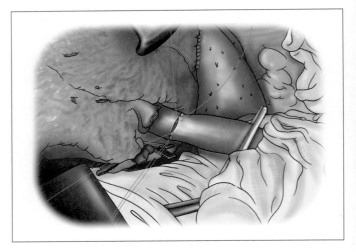

- 아랫쪽까지 온 실을 바깥으로 통과시키되 아랫쪽에 미리 tagging해둔 suture와 tie하지는 않는다. Backward로 두어번 running suture를 시행한 뒤 rubber shot으로 잡아두고 당겨둔다.

- 윗쪽의 남은 실을 이용하여 아래쪽으로 running suture를 시행한다. 세 땀 정도 남겨둔 상태에서 anastomosis distal을 bulldog clamp로 잡아둔뒤, proximal side에 clamping 될 iliac clamp를 일시적으로 풀어서 congestion 된 blood를 빼주고 air가 없어지도록 한다. 그리고 iliac clamp로 다시 잡아두며, heparin을 lumen 내부에 넣어 혈전이 생기지 않도록 한다.

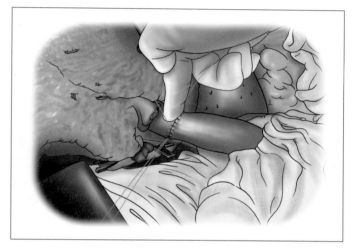

- 나머지 running suture를 시행한 뒤에 vein diameter의 1.5배 정도의 간격의 growth factor를 둔 채로 tie를 여섯 차례 시행한다.

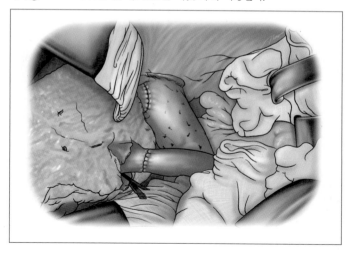

- RHV를 잡고 있던 Satinsky clamp를 풀고, portal vein의 iliac clamp와 bulldog clamp를 풀어서 reperfusion을 시행한다.
- Reperfusion 직후 warm saline으로 irrigation 및 warming을 시행하며 anastomosis 쪽에 bleeding control을 수행한다.

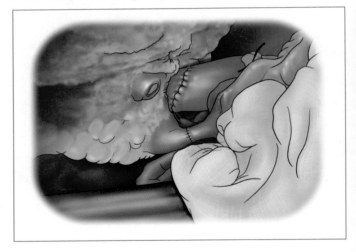

- Hepatic artery anastomosis는 적절한 flow, 적절한 tension, 그리고 intimal dissection이 없는 혈관을 이용하는 것이 중요함. Right, middle, left hepatic artery부터 hepatic artery proper까지 적절한 혈관이 없는 경우 right gastroepiploic artery 등의 extra-anatomical reconstruction까지 고려해볼 수 있다.
- 술자의 선호도에 따라 microscopic anastomosis를 할 수도 있으며, 8-0 ethilon을 이용하여 running 또는 interrupted suture로 anastomosis할 수 있다.

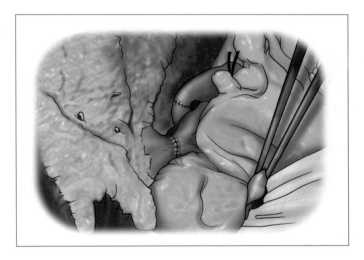

- Bile duct anastomosis를 하기 전에 leakage test를 해서 다른 opening이 있는지 확인한다.
- 6-0 Prolene이나 6-0 PDS를 사용한다. Interrupted suture로 앞뒤 모두 하거나, posterior running, anterior interrupted로 할 수도 있으며 duct가 큰 경우 모두 running suture를 시행하기도 한다.
- Multiple duct opening에 작은 duct가 있는 경우 silicon stent를 넣고 absorbable suture로 고정하기도 한다.

In case of pre-transplantation portal vein thrombosis

Portal vein thrombosis can be classified based on Yerdel's grade.

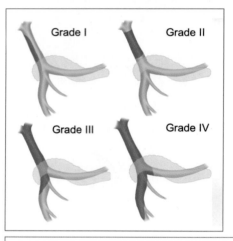

Grade I

<50% thrombosis of PV

with or without minimal extension to SMV

Grade II

>50% occlusion of PV, including total occlusion,

 with or without minimal extension to SMC

Grade III

Complete thrombosis of both PV and

proximal SMV while distal SMV is patent

Grade IV

Complete thrombosis of the PV and

proximal and distal SMV

To achieve sufficient portal inflow is vital for the success of liver transplantation. In case of portal vein thrombosis identified preoperatively, thorough planning is required. It is best to perform successful thrombectomy and anastomose with the recipient's native portal vein. Even with successful thrombectomy, collateral shunt ligation can be necessary to prevent steal syndrome to the liver. However, when portal flow in insufficient despite thrombectomy, extra-anatomical portal reconstruction using a jump graft can be an alternative. SMV can be the first option for jump graft inflow while other inflow such as left renal vein can be used when splenorenal shunt is present.

(1) Eversion thrombectomy ± collateral shunt ligation (First choice)

(2) Extra-anatomical reconstruction using Jump graft

① Inflow from SMV, splenic vein or enlarged collaterals such as coronary vein

② In case of mesenteric-systemic shunt formation, systemic veins such as left renal vein can be used. (ex. Splenorenal shunt)

③ Cryopreserved iliac veins can be used for jump graft. However, meticulous surgical skills are required since enlarged collaterals are highly friable and can risk the recipient with hemorrhage.

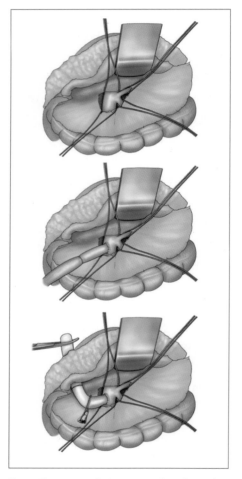

Figure. Extra-anatomical reconstruction of portal vein using jump graft from superior mesenteric vein.

CHAPTER 08.

POST-TRANSPLANT MANAGEMENT

I. Recipient Management - Immediate Postoperative care at ICU

1. Fluid management

1) Urine output: Consider preoperative renal function, intraoperative volume status, anhepatic time, and functional status of the liver graft. Wait for recovery from oliguria rather than manipulate, first. The excessive fluid challenge can cause pulmonary edema.

2) Central venous pressure: under 10 mmHg

3) Central Pontine Myelinolysis (CPM) caution

   (1) Hyponatremia should be corrected at a rate of no more than 10 mmol/L of sodium per 2 day/ 4 mmol/L per hr

(2) If rapidly corrected, lower the sodium level again

(3) Aggressive management of postoperative hyperosmolarity due to hyperglycemia and possibly uremia

2. Transfusion

1) Red Blood Cells

(1) Pre-storage leukocyte reduced RBC

(2) Target : Hematocrit 30, Hemoglobin 8-10

(3) Indication : Hemoglobin below 7 g/dl

2) Platelet

(1) Leukocyte-depleted platelet concentrate (LD-PC), Single donor platerlet (SDP)

(2) Indication : PLT < 30,000

3) Cryoprecipitate

(1) Indication : fibrinogen < 100

4) Fresh Frozen Plasma

(1) First of all, wait long enough for graft function recovery

(2) If necessary, consult with professors or fellows

(3) Indication : PT INR > 3.0

(4) In children: Do not give any procoagulants (FFP, cryoprecipitates, platelets, or Vit. K) routinely due to thrombosis risk

5) Albumin, insurance coverage

(1) < 3.0   : cover 1pack /1day

(2) 3.1~3.4 : only 100/100

(3) > 3.5   : do not cover.

3. Nutritional management

1) EN : 이식 전 – 정상식이 진행중 목표열량의 50%미만 섭취가 1주이상 지속된 환자가 Enteral route를 통한 feeding이 가능한 경우

   이식 후 – Child B or C 환자 중 enteral route feeding이 가능한 경우

2) PN : 3일 이내 oral diet 및 enteral route diet가 불가능 할 것으로 판단될 경우

3) Supplement의 'Nutrition protocol' 참조

4. Other medications

1) Prostaglandin E (PGE, Prostandin®, PGE1 or Eglandin®, PGE10)

   (1) Period of use: after reperfusion - POD#4, total 8

   (2) Usage: Prostandin® 35 A bid (8회), Eglandin® 75 A bid (8회) (≥60 kg) Prostandin® 25 A bid (8회), Eglandin® 50 A bid (8회) (>60 kg)

   (3) Remove central line after PGE infusion (POD#5, transfer to GW)

2) Nafamostat

   (1) Period of use: after reperfusion – POD#6, total 7

   (2) Usage: 300 mg (6 vial) in 5DW 50 mL, ivs 2 cc/hr

3) Dalteparin- Low Molecular heparin

   (1) Period of use: after HA anastomosis finish - POD#6, total 7

   (2) Usage: 3000 IU qd in ≥ 60 kg, 2500 IU qd in <60 kg

4) Antithrombin III

   (1) Period of use: - POD#9 (LDLT) / - POD#6 (DDLT)

   (2) Usage: Antithrombin III 500unit, ivs q 6hr for 10 days (Adult)

   Antithrombin III 100 unit ivs q 6hrs for 7 days (Child)

    5) Aspirin, only adult LDLT

        (1) Period of use: from POD#5~

        (2) Usage: aspirin coated 100 mg p.o. qd

    6) Lenograstim, granulocyte colony-stimulating factor (G-CSF)

        (1) Indication & insurance coverage: absolute neutrophil count (ANC)<1000

        (2) Usage: lenograstim 100 mg(<50 kg) or 250 mg(>50 kg) iv or sc

        (3) Target: ANC > 2000

    7) Time of taking pills

Medication	Time	Description
Esomeprazole	7A (T07)	With immunosuppressant
Steroids	8A/6P (2W)	Immediately after meal
Entecavir	7A (T07)	With immunosuppressant
Itraconazole – Syrup	7A/8P (Q12)	With immunosuppressant
Itraconazole – Capsule	8A/6P (2W)	
TMP-SMX	WM	Immediately after meal
UDCA 2T	8A/6P (2W)	Immediately after meal
Diuretics	8A/6P (WM or 2W)	Immediately after meal

5. Postoperative examinations

    1) Doppler ultrasonography

        (1) At POD#1,3,(5),7

        (2) Checkpoints (Check Supplement)

Inflow (Portal vein, Allograft vein, Hepatic artery) and outflow (hepatic vein)
RI (Resistive index) of hepatic artery (peak systolic velocity - end diastolic velocity)/peak systolic velocity
Liver echogenicity
Fluid collection and hematoma formation

(3) Consider further exam include liver CT scan if needed

- Postoperative AST or ALT > 1000, or AST or ALT increase > 2 folds

2) Liver CT, Hepatobiliary scintigraphy (DISIDA)

(1) At POD#14

(2) JP No.2, placed at the hilum should be removed after confirmation of CT and DISIDA.

3) Liver fibroscan

(1) Around POD#14~#21 and 3 months

4) Chest X-ray

(1) Daily check at ICU

II. Recipient management - Early Postoperative care at ward(sub-ICU)

1. Sustained Ascites

1) Doppler USG f/u: especially HV (r/o HVOO)

2) Consider Diuretics (Furosemide, Spironolactone) or Propranolol administration

2. Sustained Hyperbilirubinemia

1) r/o biliary complication vs. r/o graft dysfunction

2) Examinations

(1) Doppler US f/u: intrahepatic duct dilatation or fluid collection

(2) Liver CT

(3) DISIDA

(4) Biopsy: consultation with professors

III. Management of Readmitted recipient

1. Timing of Allograft dysfunction

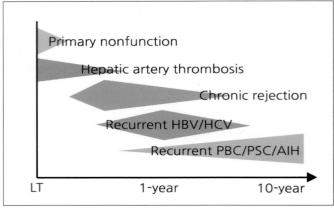

(Rosen, Clin Liver Dis 2000; 4:675-689)

2. Disease Recurrence After OLT (Kotlyar et al., Am J Gastroenterol 2006;101:1370)

Etiology of disease	Recurrence rate
Hepatitis C	>90% (needs more data with the advent of DAA)
Hepatitis B	<5% with prophylaxis
Hepatocellular carcinoma	8-15%
Primary biliary cirrhosis	11-23%
Primary sclerosing cholangitis	9-47%
Autoimmune hepatitis	16-46%
Alcoholic cirrhosis	<5%
Nonalcoholic steatohepatitis	11-38%

3. Evaluation

1) Cause of Readmission

    (1) Elevation of AST/ALT

    (2) Elevation of total Bilirubin

    (3) Infection: Fever, CMV antigenemia, Herpes Zoster

    (4) R/O Recurrence of primary disease

    (5) R/O PTLD or other malignancy

    (6) Others: Nutritional problem

    (7) For intervention (PTBD or ERCP)

    (8) For Immunosuppressant change

2) Operation date

3) Primary Cause of LT

    (1) HCC: Alpha-fetoprotein, Recent Liver CT

    (2) HBV-related

        ① Current medication (HBIG/Lamivudine/Adefovir⋯)

        ② HBsAg/anti-HBs titer

        ③ HBV DNA Quantitation

        ④ HBV YMDD mutation (in case of recurrence)

    (3) HCV-related

        ① HCV RNA Quantitation

        ② HCV genotype

4) Operative procedures

    (1) Deceased / Living Donor LT

    (2) Duct reconstruction: Hepaticojejunostomy / Duct-to-duct anastomosis

        ① Single/double, stent usage

② PTBD indwelling: route and tip placement

(3) HA, HV, PV reconstructions

5) Previous problems

: history of previous intervention

6) Recent laboratory or radiologic findings

: CBC, LFT, CRP, CMV antigenemia, Doppler US, Liver CT

4. Examinations of readmitted patient with abnormal LFT

1) Differential diagnosis

(1) R/O Biliary complication, R/O Cholangitis

(2) R/O Primary disease recur

① Viral hepatitis, Autoimmune hepatitis, HCC

② R/O HBV recur, R/O HCV active replication

(3) R/O Rejection, R/O Graft failure

(4) R/O Viral Infection

2) Examinations

(1) CBC with diff. LFT with D-Bil, GGT, CRP, AFP(HCC)

(2) Doppler US: HA/PV/HV/Bile duct evaluation

(3) Liver CT

① R/O Perihepatic Fluid collection

② R/O Bile duct dilatation

③ R/O insufficient perfusion

(4) DISIDA

① R/O Biliary leakage

② R/O Biliary obstruction

③ R/O hepatic dysfunction

(5) Culture (Ordinary bacteria and fungus): Blood, Urine, Sputum, Bile (PTBD), Ascites (PCD)

(6) PTBD re-check (PTBD indwelling)

(7) Hepatitis profile/HBV DNA Quan./HBV YMDD mutation (HBsAg (+)일때)

(8) HCV RNA Detection /Quan. (PCR)

(9) CMV antigenemia

(10) EBV PCR (high-risk recipient)

(11) FANA, Quan./Smooth Muscle Antibodies/Mitochondrial Antibodies

(12) Biopsy

　　① R/O Acute Rejection vs. Graft failure (chronic rejection)

　　② R/O Hepatitis (HBV, HCV)

　　③ R/O viral infection - CMV, EBV, HSV

Biopsy in liver transplant recipients

Biopsy examination with

✓ C4d

✓ PRA screening HLA class Ⅰ, Ⅱ (BL5247)

PRA screening examination (+),

✓ "Preop specimen"PRA screening (specimen - P35 liver)

✓ Comment "Preop specimen"

If PRA screening examination (+),

✓ HLA Ab Single Identification, PRA (Class Ⅰ)

✓ HLA Ab Single Identification, PRA (Class Ⅱ)

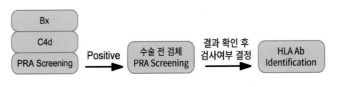

5. Management

1) Examination: Doppler USG, DISIDA, CT

2) Biopsy

    (1) If scheduled, available at admission day

    Midnight NPO→admit before noon, check PT & aPTT →consult

    biopsy

3) ERCP

    (1) Usually scheduled at OPD

    (2) Antiplatelets are discontinued 1 week before admission

    (3) Prevention: Ulinastatin 100000 unit (1 ample) in 5%DW 100 cc

mix iv q 12hrs

(4) Diet

① Procedure day– NPO

② Post-procedure day 1- diet after checking serum amylase, lipase level

4) PTBD or angiographic intervention

5) PTBD removal after Hepaticojejunostomy conversion op

: HJ conversion op ⇨ after 3 months, cholangiography ⇨ PTBD removal

6) Laboratory exams for ERBD, PTBD, T-tube removal, I-tube removal patients

: CBC, LFT, electrolyte, T-bil/D-bil, ALP/GGT, BUN/Cr, PT/aPTT

IV. Postoperative infection control: discharge education program

1. Post-LT 환자는(both LDLT/DDLT) 퇴원 전에 감염내과 협진 시행

2. Discharge education program.

1) 일상생활에서 잦은 손 씻기(외출 후, 식사 전/음식 준비 시, 흙/동물/오염환경 노출 후 등)

2) 호흡기 질환자가 있는 공간, 밀집된 공간, 공사장/축사/창고 등 먼지가 많은 공간은 가능한 한 피하고, 불가피한 경우 마스크 착용. 이식 이후 6개월간은 특히 주의를 요함.

3) 대중목욕탕, 워터파크 등 여러 사람이 사용하는 물, 지하실 등 습기가 높은 공간, 계곡/바다 수영도 가능한 피할 것.

4) 물은 끓여 먹고, 계란/육류/해산물(특히 굴, 조개)은 충분히 익혀서 섭취. 과일과 야채는 익히지 않고 섭취가 가능하나 흐르는 물에 깨끗이 세척해야 하며, 부페나 샐러드 바 등 여러 사람이 이용하여 위생을 보장하기 어려운 경우에는 섭취를 피함.

5) 반드시 금연, 금주 필요

6) 기존 사육하던 반려물을 키우는 것이 금지되는 것은 아니나, 반려동물에 대한 철저한 예방접종 및 위생관리가 필요. 예방접종에 관해서는 수의사와 상의가 필요하며 예방접종 직후에는 코/구강/분변에 대한 접촉을 피해야 함. 유기 동물을 새로 들여오는 것은 금지되며, 새장/분변 청소는 피해야 함(불가피할 경우 반드시 마스크와 장갑 착용). 파충류, 병아리, 오리, 설치류, 해외 수입동물 등은 사육하지 않는 것이 바람직함.

7) 건강보조식품은 섭취를 피하는 것이 바람직함.

V. Elevated creatinine level patients, considerations

1. Antibiotics, antiviral agent, Septrin (reduction - 3times a week[Mon,Wed,Fri])
2. CNI
3. Diuretics
4. Nephrology consultation
5. Old age, sarcopenic patients: check cystatin-C level

VI. After POD#30, consider adding of Certican® (Everolimus)

: especially HCC recipients, but Professors will decide whether to change

VII. At the time of ganciclovir treatment, beware of cytopenia and acute kidney injury

VIII. Patient with AKI : be careful of using entecavir or tenofovir for HBV

- check creatinine clearance and dose adjustment is needed

A. Out-Patient follow-up

: check blood pressure of every patient

1. Routine Lab

1) CBC with diff.

2) Chemistry profile, Electrolyte profile, Bilirubin, Direct, GGT, CRP

3) CMV antigenemia: 3개월까지만

4) Hepatitis profile

5) AFP, PIVKA-II (HCC)

6) Drug level (TDM)

7) HbA1c, Lipid profile q 3 months

2. Virus Related

1) HBV-related

HBV DNA quantitation: every 1 year

2) HCV-related

HCV RNA quantitation: every 1 year

HCV reactivation → Hepatology consultation

3. Image study

1) Non-HCC

    (1) ~ 이식후 1년까지: doppler 3개월 간격

    (2) 1Yr이후 ~: doppler와 CT- yearly, by turns

2) HCC

    (1) ~ 이식후 1년까지: CT 3개월 간격

    (2) 1Yr ~ 5Yr: CT 4개월 간격

    (3) 5Yr 이후: CT yearly

4. Postoperative 1-year exam

Examinations
Tumor marker (AFP, PIVKA, CEA, CA19-9, CA125, PSA)
UA c micro
Autoimmune lab (FANA, AMA, SMA, IgG)
Lipid profile
Mammography, routine bilateral (Female)
Bone Densitometry. (L-spine AP, Lat & Femur AP)
EGD, Colonoscopy
Liver fibroscan
PRA screening, HLA I&II (양성 시 single Identification)

5. National 5-cancer screening

	Examinations	Period
Gastric	EGD	2yrs
Colorectal	Colonoscopy	2yrs
Breast	Mammography, routine bilateral (Female)	2yrs
Gynecology	Cervical smear-> OBGY consult	2yrs
Hepatocellular	Liver USG and CT	

6. Medication

기본 medication

	Usage	Duration
Bactrim	1T qd (WM) :daily	- 6months
Esomeprazole	20 mg qd (T07)	Discontinue with MPD (postop 3month)
Diogel	입원 중 1일 3회: 3PRN(아침, 저녁, 취침전) 퇴원 후 1일 2회: MHS(아침, 취침전)	
Aspirin coated	1T (100 mg) qd (WM)	Lifelong
UDCA	2T bid (2W)	Lifelong

1) HTN in LT

   (1) Prevalence: more than 50% after LT

   (2) Cause if HTN after LT:

      ① Systemic vasoconstriction after LT (vasodilated status before LT)

      ② Endothelin-1 (potent vasoconstrictor) elevated in first few days after LT

      ③ Calcineurin inhibitos: vasoconstrictors↑ (endothelin, thromboxane) vasodilators↓ (NO, prostacyclin) Sodium and water retention

      ④ Steroid: Sodium and water retention

      ⑤ Loss of normal nocturnal BP decrease: normalizes 1-2 years in 50%.

   (3) No proteinuria: CCB (Amlodipine)

   (4) Proteinuria : ACE inhibitor or ARB

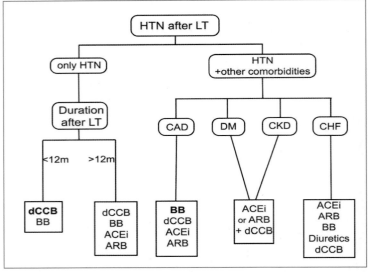

(Najeed et al., Int J Cardiol 2011 Oct 6;152(1):4-6)

2) DM medication in LT

   (1) Oral hypoglycemic agents (OHA): sulfonylurea, a-glucosidase
      inhibitor

   (2) Insulin

      ① intermediate-acting: NPH

      ② long-acting: glarnine, detemir

3) Dyslipidemia - statin 계열 약물

7. Vaccination: 3장 Infection part참조

: 이식 전 vaccination이 시행되지 못한 경우 및 추가 접종은 이식 3개월 후 clinically stable할 때 시행. 단, influenza vaccination은 유행시기를 놓칠 수 있으므로 이식 1개월 후부터 접종 가능(according to the AST guidline)

8. OPD follow-up period

1) postop 1 month: every 2 week
2) 1 month – 1 yr : every 4-5 weeks
3) After 1yr: every 2-3 months

CHAPTER 09.

LIVER TRANSPLANTATION PROTOCOL

I. Pre-Op. Order (POD#-1)

1. V/S q 8 hr
2. W/A
3. NPO from the evening
4. Check I/O q 8hr
5. Check BWt.
6. Check BST q6hr (if<200, q12hr)
7. Get Op Permission
8. 0.1% Chlorohexidine Gargling q 6hr
9. Apply DVT prophylaxis (antiembolic cuff prep to OR)
10. Check Lab(입원 전에 tumor marker, viral marker 시행되어 있고 1개월 이내라면 재시행 하지 않아도 됩니다.)
11. Check HLA-tying(전에 안 했을 시에)
12. Check HCC image w/u (1달 이내의 것이 없으면 fellow 컨펌받고 CT)
13. Antibiotics skin test: Cefotaxime, ampicillin/sulbactam
14. Allow self-medication: HTN meds, Thyroid meds.

15. Prep to OR (ampicillin/sulbactam 3 g x 2, cefotaxime 2 gX2/Basiliximab /HBIG / MPD / Nafamostat & Alprostadil (only LDLT)/ 5% albumin (only DDLT)

16. 5% DNK1 1 L iv with 80 cc/hr

17. Famotidine 20 mg + NS 50 mL mivs

18. Phazyme 2T p.o. qd

19. Magcorol 250 mL (1B) p.o. bid

20. HBIG 10,000 IU: HBV related or Anti-HBc (+) donor (prep to OR)

21. Esp) HBIG 20,000 IU: HBV DNA or HBe Ag (+) Recipient (prep to OR)

22. Basiliximab 20 mg (prep to OR)

23. Methylprednisolone 500 mg (prep to OR)

24. Nafamostat 50 mg (prep to OR): LDLT only

25. Alprostadil 100 mcg (prep to OR): LDLT only

26. 5% Albumin 250 mL X2 (prep to OR): DDLT only

27. Chest PA

28. CBC with Diff., Chemistry profile, Electrolyte, Ammonia, TCO2, Amylase/Lipase, PT/aPTT, AFP, CEA, NT-proBNP, CRP

29. HBeAg, Anti-HBe Ab, HBV DNA Quan.(PCR)

    A.   HCV-RNA detection, HBV drug resistance mutation

    B.   Antithrombin III activity, fibrinogen, PIVKA-II

30. For patient with HCV, HCV genotype, HCV RNA Quantitation

31. HLA crossmatch, HLA crossmatch (DDLT 시행안함)

    HLA-A, B typing (DNA), HLA-DR Typing (DNA), PRA screening, HLA class I, II

32. Blood culture *3 with fungus culture

33. Gram stain and Culture (Urine, Sputum, stool, throat swab)

34. Fungus culture (Urine, Sputum, stool, throat swab)

35. Gram stain and Culture: Nasal swab –MRSA, Rectal swab-VRE

36. Stool exam & Occult blood

Ⅱ. PreOp. Order (Op day)

1. V/S q 8hr
2. WA
3. NPO
4. Check body weight
5. Allow self-medication : HTN, Thyroid meds.
6. Prep to OR (L-tube, antiembolic cuff, medication)
7. Check antibiotics (cefotaxim 2 g TID, ampicillin/sulbactam 3 g QID)
8. Plasma solution 1 L iv with 80cc/hr
9. Cefotaxime 2 g x 3 (total 6 g)
10. Ampicillin/sulbactam 3 g x 4 (total 12 g)
11. Famotidine 20 mg + 5%DW 50mL mivs
12. Intra OP sono preparation (pediatric is essential) and arrange
   * No need for consultating department of radiology for intra-op sonography in DDLT (Except pediatric LT)

Ⅲ.Post-Op Order

(Op day)

1. V/S q 15min until stable/then q 30min x 4/then q 1hr
   : Warming to maintain core temp>36'C
2. BR
3. NPO
4. I/O q 4hr (hourly urine check : <1 cc/kg/hr → notify to Dr.)
5. CVP monitoring q 6hr
6. Keep A-line with continuous monitoring
   Notifiy to Dr. if MAP < 65 mmHg or SBP > 160 mmHg
7. Check Bwt daily
8. Keep Foley in situ & JP drains to closed drainage
9. L-tube aspiration q 4hr & postural drainage
10. Position change q 2hr
11. Line change : every 4 days
12. Ventilator care
    - HOB 30°
    - DVT prophylaxis IPC
    - Stress ulcer drug prophylaxis
    - Pain assess q 8 hrs
    - Apply restraint when is ir nore than RASS +1
13. Remifentanil start from 0.05 mcg/kg/min
14. BST check q 6hr
    : If BGL <100 or >240, △BGL >80

⇨ recheck 2hrs later
1) **Initiation**
   (1) 160 mg/dl< BGL < 240 mg/dl ⇨ starting rate: 1unit/hr
   (2) 240 mg/dl < BGL ⇨ starting rate: 2unit/hr
2) ** Maintenance**
   (1) BGL BGL < 100 ⇨ stop for 2hrs & notify & restart when >180 by rate -1unit/hr
   (2) 100 ≤ BGL < 140 ⇨ rate -1units/hr
   (3) 140 ≤ BGL < 160 ⇨ maintain rate
   (4) 160≤ BGL < 240 ⇨ rate +1unit/hr (maintain if BGL is decreasing)
   (5) 240 ≤ BGL < 300 ⇨ rate +2unit/hr (maintain if BGL is decreasing)
   (6) 300 ≤ BGL ⇨ rate +2unit/hr & notify
15. 0.1% Chlorohexidine Gargling q 6hr
16. 10% dextrose 40 cc/hr +Tamipool 1 vial
17. Alprostadil 700 mcg bid (5DW 50 mL) ⇨ CIV 4 cc/hr (< 60 kg, 500 mcg bid)
18. Nafamostat 300 mg (5DW 50 mL) ⇨ CIV 2 cc/hr
19. Dalteparin 3,000 IU (5DW 50 mL) ⇨ CIV 2 cc/hr : Living or split only (<60 kg, 2,500 IU)

20. Anti-Thrombin III 500 IU (in 5dw 50 mL) IVS q 6hr (LDLT POD#9, DDLT POD#7까지)
21. Cefotaxime 2 g ivs q 8hr
22. Ampicillin/sulbactam 3 g (in 5DW 50 mL) ivs q 6hr
23. Ambroxol 15 mg ivs q 6hr
24. Famotidine 20 mg + 5dw 50 mL mivs q 12hr
25. Vit. K 10 mg + 5DW50cc miv q 24hr
26. HBIG 10,000 IU + 5%DW 200mL : HBV related recipient or Anti-HBc (+) Donor - 1주일만 투여HBIG 20,000 IU dose standard: HBV DNA(+) or HBe Ag(+)
27. Glutathione 600 mg + NS 100 mL mivs q 12hr
28. Itraconazole syrup 100mg bid: during NPO
29. Diogel 1p bid
30. Remifentanil 0.05 mcg/kg/min civ (when using a ventilator)
31. prn) norepinephrine 0.05 mcg/kg/min CIV
32. CBC, eletrolyte, chemistry, PT/aPTT/fibrinogen, D-bil, r-GT, LDH, Mg, Ionized Ca, S-osm, ABGA, Anti-Thrombin III, FDP, ammonia, UA c micro, amylase, lipase, chest AP(p), EKG(p)
33. CBC, electrolyte, PT/aPTT/fibrinogen, T-bil/AST/ALT, q 6hr

POD # 0 저녁	Alprostadil 1 Dalteparin 1 Nafamostat 1	
POD # 1	Alprostadil 2 Dalteparin 1 Nafamostat 1	MMF start, Doppler Confirm antiviral agent prescription POD#1 SOW (EN 20cc/hr for high MELD)
POD # 2,3	Same as above	POD#2 SFD (EN 40cc/hr for high MELD) POD # 3 FK start,Doppler
POD # 4	Alprostadil 1 (total 8) Dalteparin 1 Nafamostat 1	SBD (EN 60cc/hr to target kcal for high MELD) POD#4 SBD even high MELD
POD # 5	Dalteparin 1 Nafamostat 1 C-line removal	Aspirin, SMX-TMP start Doppler
POD# 6	Dalteparin 1 Nafamostat 1	
POD# 7		Doppler
POD#14		CT, DISIDA, Fibroscan

Ⅳ. LT POD #1

1. V/S q 1hr: warming to maintain core temp>36'C
2. BR
3. L-tube removal & SOW (L-tube 유지하는 경우: natural drainage)
4. I/O q 8hr (hourly urine check: <1 cc/kg/hr → notify to Dr.)
5. CVP monitoring q 6hr
6. Keep A-line with continuous monitoring
   Notifiy to Dr. if MAP < 65 mmHg or SBP < 160 mmHg
7. Check Body weight daily
8. Keep Foley in situ & JP drains to closed drainage
9. Position change q 2hr
10. Check (culture POD#1,3,5)
11. Pain assessment q 8hr
12. Daily abdominal sterile dressing change
13. BST check q 6hr
    : If BGL <100 or >240, △BGL >80 ⇨ recheck 2hrs later
    1) **Initiation**
       (1) 160 mg/dl< BGL < 240 mg/dl ⇨ starting rate: 1unit/hr
       (2) 240 mg/dl < BGL ⇨ starting rate: 2unit/hr
    2) ** Maintenance**
       (1) BGL BGL < 100 ⇨ stop for 2hrs & notify & restart when >180 by rate -1unit/hr
       (2) 100 ≤ BGL < 140 ⇨ rate -1units/hr
       (3) 140 ≤ BGL < 160 ⇨ maintain rate
       (4) 160 ≤ BGL < 240 ⇨ rate +1unit/hr (maintain if BGL is decreasing)
       (5) 240 ≤ BGL < 300 ⇨ rate +2unit/hr (maintain if BGL is decreasing)
       (6) 300 ≤BGL ⇨ rate +2unit/hr & notify
14. 0.1% Chlorohexidine Gargling q 6hr
15. 5%DW 1 L 40 cc/hr + Tamipool 1 vial

16. Alprosdtadil 700 mcg bid (5DW 50 mL) ⇨ CIV 4 cc/hr (< 60 kg, 500 mcg bid)

17. Nafamostat 300 mg (5DW 50 mL) ⇨ CIV 2 cc/hr

18. Dalteparin 3,000 IU (5DW 50 mL) ⇨ CIV 2 cc/hr : Living or split only (<60 kg, 2,500 IU)

19. Anti-Thrombin III 500 IU (in 5dw 50 mL) ivs q 6hr (LDLT POD#9, DDLT POD#7까지)

20. Cefotaxime 2 g ivs q 8hr

21. Ampicillin/ sulbactam 3 g (in 5DW 50mL) ivs q 6hr

22. MMF 750 mg bid (MEDL 25이상일 경우는 POD#3일 500 bid로 시작)

23. Methylprednisolone 500 mg (in 5% DW 50 mL) ivs qd

24. HBIG 10,000 IU/20,000 IU + 5%DW 200 mL

25. Itraconazole 100 mg bid (syrup,during NPO)

26. Ambroxol 15 mg ivs q 6hr

27. Famotidine 20 mg + 5% DW 50 mL mivs q 12hr

28. Vit. K 10 mg + 5DW 50 cc miv q 24hr

29. Glutathione 600 mg + NS 100 mL mivs q 12hr

30. L-arginine HCL 15 g +NS 100 ml mivs q 12hr (POD#7까지)

31. Diomagnite 3.8 g bid

32. PRN) quetiapine 25 mg HS. (insomnia)

33. chemistry, fibrinogen, D-bil, r-GT, LDH, Mg, Ion Ca, S-osm, amylase, lipase, ammonia, UA c micro, CRP, ABGA

34. T-bil/AST/ALT q 6 hr

35. CBC, e, PT/aPTT q 12 hr

36. Chest AP (p), EKG (p),

37. Gram stain culture & fungus culture: Blood (x2), JP (x3), urine, TTA

38. CMV antigenemia (Mon, Wed, Fri)

39. Liver Doppler sono (portable)

40. If HBsAg (+) ⇨ antiviral agent (이전 복용대로 처방)

41. Pain control. prn) hydromorphone 1 mg. if NRS > 4.

42. Delirium control. Consider prn) dexmedetomidine 0.2 mcg/kg/hr CIV if RASS > +2

V. LT POD #2

1. V/S q 1hr: warming to maintain core temp>36'C
2. BR
3. SFD ⇨ EN feeding 40 cc/hr for high MELD greater than MELD 25
4. I/O q 8hr (hourly urine check: <1 cc/kg/hr → notify to Dr.)
5. CVP monitoring q 6hr
6. Keep A-line with continuous monitoring
   Notifiy to Dr. if MAP < 65 mmHg or SBP < 160 mmHg
7. Check Bwt daily
8. Keep Foley in situ & JP drains to closed drainage
9. Position change q 2hr
10. Line change: every 4 days
11. BST check q 6hr

    : If BGL <100 or >240, △BGL >80 ⇨ recheck 2hrs later

    1) **Initiation**

    (1) 160 mg/dl< BGL < 240 mg/dl ⇨ starting rate: 1unit/hr

    (2) 240 mg/dl < BGL ⇨ starting rate: 2unit/hr

    2) ** Maintenance**

    (1) BGL < 100 ⇨ stop for 2hrs & notify & restart when >180 by rate -1unit/hr

    (2) 100 ≤ BGL < 140 ⇨ rate -1units/hr

    (3) 140 ≤ BGL < 160 ⇨ maintain rate

    (4) 160 ≤ BGL < 240 ⇨ rate +1unit/hr (maintain if BGL is decreasing)

    (5) 240 ≤ BGL < 300 ⇨ rate +2unit/hr (maintain if BGL is decreasing)

    (6) 300≤ BGL ⇨ rate +2unit/hr & notify

12. 0.1% Chlorohexidine Gargling q 6hr
13. 5% DW 1L 40 cc/hr +Tamipool 1 vial
14. Alprosdtadil 700 mcg bid (5DW 50 mL) ⇨ CIV 4 cc/hr (< 60 kg, 500 mcg bid)
15. Nafamostat 300 mg (5DW 50 mL) ⇨ CIV 2 cc/hr
16. Dalteparin 3,000 IU (5DW 50 mL) ⇨ CIV 2 cc/hr : Living or split only (<60 kg,

2,500 IU)

17. Anti-Thrombin III 500 IU (in 5dw 50 mL) ivs q 6hr (LDLT POD#9, DDLT POD#7까지)

18. Cefotaxime 2 g ivs q 8hr

19. Ampicillin/sulbactam 3 g (in 5DW 50 mL) ivs q 6hr

20. Methylprednisolone 250 mg (in 5%DW 50 mL) ivs qD

21. MMF 750 mg bid

22. HBIG 10,000 IU/20,000 IU + 5%DW 200cc mivs

23. Itraconazole capsule 100 mg bid

24. Ambroxol 15 mg ivs q 6hr

25. Famotidine 20 mg + 5DW 50 mL mivs q 12hr

26. Vit. K 10 mg + 5DW50cc miv q 24hr

27. Glutathione 600 mg in N/S100 mL miv q 12hr

28. L-arginine HCL 15 g +NS 100 mL mivs q 12hr

29. PRN) quetiapine 25 mg HS

30. ABGA, chemistry, fibrinogen (q12hr), D-bil, r-GT, LDH, Mg, Ion Ca, S-osm, ammonia, UA c micro, amylase, lipase, CRP

31. T-bil/AST/ALT q 6hr

32. CBC, e', PT/aPTT q 6hr

33. Chest AP(p)

34. CMV antigenemia (Mon, Wed, Fri)

35. If HBsAg (+) ⇨ antiviral agent (이전 복용대로 처방)

36. Pain control. Prn) hydromorphone 1 mg. if NRS > 4

37. Delirium control. Consider prn) dexmedetomidine 0.2 mcg/kg/hr CIV If RASS > +2

38. Gram stain & culture (femoral sheath tip)

39. Diomagnite 3.8 g bid

VI. LT POD #3

1. V/S q 1hr: warming to maintain core temp>36'C
2. BR
3. SBD ⇨ EN feeding 60 cc/hr to target kcal for high MELD greater than MELD 25
4. I/O q 8hr (hourly urine check: <1 cc/kg/hr → notify to Dr.)
5. CVP monitoring q 6hr, Keep A-line with continuous monitoring
6. Nofify to Dr if MAP < 65 mmHg or SBP < 160
7. Check Bwt
8. Keep Foley in situ & JP drains to closed drainage
9. abdominal sterile dressing change
10. BST check q 6hr (EN feeding시)

    : If BGL <100 or >240, △BGL >80 ⇨ recheck 2hrs later

    1) **Initiation**

    (1) 160 mg/dl< BGL < 240 mg/dl ⇨ starting rate: 1unit/hr

    (2) 240 mg/dl < BGL ⇨ starting rate: 2unit/hr

    2) ** Maintenance**

    (1) BGL < 100 ⇨ stop for 2hrs & notify & restart when >180 by rate -1unit/hr

    (2) 100 ≤ BGL < 140 ⇨ rate -1units/hr

    (3) 140 ≤ BGL < 160 ⇨ maintain rate

    (4) 160 ≤ BGL < 240 ⇨ rate +1unit/hr (maintain if BGL is decreasing)

    (5) 240 ≤ BGL < 300 ⇨ rate +2unit/hr (maintain if BGL is decreasing)

    (6) 300 ≤ BGL ⇨ rate +2unit/hr & notify

    BST check q6hr(SBD)

    BSL 200~250 : RI 4U SC

    BSL 251~300 : RI 8U SC

    BSL 301~350 : RI 12U SC

    BSL>350 or <80 : notify to Dr

11. 0.1% Chlorohexidine Gargling q 6hr
12. 5% DW 1L 40cc/hr +Tamipool 1 vial

13. Alprosdtadil 700 mcg bid (5DW 50 mL) ⇨ CIV 4cc/hr (< 60 kg, 500 mcg bid)

14. Nafamostat 300 mg (5DW 50 mL) ⇨ CIV 2cc/hr

15. Dalteparin 3,000 IU (5DW 50mL) ⇨ CIV 2cc/hr : Living or split only (<60 kg, 2,500 IU)

16. Anti-Thrombin III 500 IU (in 5dw 50 mL) ivs q 6hr (LDLT POD#9, DDLT POD#7까지)

17. Tacrolimus ( ) mg p.o. at 8 PM (start)

18. MMF 750 mg bid

19. Methylprednisolone 125 mg (in 5DW 50 mL) ivs qd

20. Esomeprazol 20 mg p.o. qd

21. Itraconazole capsule 100 mg bid

22. Diomagnite 3.8 g bid

23. UDCA: POD#3 start, 200 mg p.o. bid

24. PRN) 20% albumin 100cc alb <3.0

25. Vit. K 10 mg + 5DW 50cc ivs q 24hr

26. Glutathione 600 mg in NS 100 mL q 12hr

27. L-arginine HCL 15 g +NS 100 mL mivs q 12hr

28. HBIG 10,000 IU/20, 000 IU + 5%DW200 mL

29. PRN) queitapine 25 mg HS. insomnia

30. CBC, e, PT/aPTT, T-bil/AST/ALT, q 8hr

31. chemistry, fibrinogenD-bil, r-GT, LDH, Mg, Ion Ca, S-osm,

32. ammonia, UA c micro, urine (e, osm), CRP, chest AP (p)

33. Gram stain culture & fungus culture: Blood (x2), JP (x3), urine, sputum

34. CMV antigenemia (Mon, Wed, Fri)

35. Doppler US F/U

36. If HBsAg (+) ⇨ antiviral agent(이전 복용대로 처방)

37. PRN) Pain control: hydromorphone 1 mg

Ⅶ. LT POD #4

1. V/S q 1hr: warming to maintain core temp>36'C
2. BR
3. SBD (sterilized porridge)
4. I/O q 8hr (hourly urine check: <1cc/kg/hr → notify to Dr.)
5. Check Bwt daily
6. Keep Foley in situ & JP drains to closed drainage
7. Line change: every 4 days
8. BST check q 6hr

   BST check q 6hrs

   RI sliding MDI

Blood glucose	RI subcut.injection
201 - 250	4
251 - 300	8
301 - 350	12
<80 or > 350	call Dr.

9. 0.1% Chlorohexidine Gargling q 6hr
10. Main fluid d/c
11. Alprosdtadil 700 mcg qd (5DW 50 mL) ⇨ CIV 4 cc/hr (< 60 kg, 500 mcg qd)
12. Nafamostat 300 mg (5DW 50 mL) ⇨ CIV 2 cc/hr
13. Dalteparin 3,000 IU (5DW 50 mL) ⇨ CIV 2 cc/hr : Living or split only (<60 kg, 2,500 IU)
14. Anti-Thrombin III 500 IU (in 5dw 50 mL) ivs q 6hr (LDLT POD#9, DDLT POD#7 까지)
15. Basiliximab 20 mg/NS 100 cc 1V ivs
16. Tacrolimus (/) p.o. bid after confirm
17. MMF 750 mg p.o bid
18. Methylprednisolone 75 mg ivs q d
19. Esomeprazole 20 mg p.o qd

20. Itraconazole capsule 100 mg bid
21. Diomagnite 3.8 g bid
22. UDCA 200 mg p.o bid
23. Vit. K 10 mg + 5DW50cc miv qd
24. Glutathione 600 mg in NS 100 mL q 12hr
25. L-arginine HCL 15 g +NS 100 mL mivs q 12hr
26. HBIG 10,000 IU/20,000 IU + 5%DW 200 mL mivs
27. PRN) 20 % Alb 1B ivs (alb<3.0)
28. CBC, PT/aPTT, T-bil/AST/ALT, e'q 8hr
29. chemistry, fibrinogen, D-bil, r-GT, LDH, Mg, Ion Ca, S-osm, CRP, ammonia, UA c
    micro
30. Tacrolimus level
31. CMV antigenemia (Mon, Wed, Fri)
32. Chest AP (p)
33. If HBsAg (+) ⇨ antiviral agent(이전 복용대로 처방)
34. PRN) Pain control; hydromorphone
35. PRN) Quetiapine 25 mg HS p.o for insomnia
36. PRN BST SC 4u, 8u,12u, 각각

VIII. LT POD#5

1. V/S q 1hr
2. BR
3. SBD (sterilized porridge)
4. I/O q 8hr (hourly urine check: <1 cc/kg/hr → notify to Dr.)
5. Check Bwt daily
6. Keep Foley in situ & JP drains to closed drainage
7. Position change q 2hr
8. Line change: every 4 days
9. Daily abdominal sterile dressing change
10. BST check q 6hr RI sliding scale

    BST check q 6hrs

    RI sliding MDI

Blood glucose		RI subcut.injection
201 - 250	4	
251 - 300	8	
301 - 350	12	
<80 or > 350	call Dr.	

11. 0.1% Chlorohexidine Gargling q 6hr
12. start Aspirin 100 mg (Living or split DDLT) if plt > 50k
13. Nafamostat 300 mg (5DW 50 mL) ⇨ CIV 2 cc/hr
14. Dalteparin 3,000 IU (5DW 50 mL) ⇨ CIV 2 cc/hr : Living or split only (<60 kg, 2,500 IU)
15. Anti-Thrombin III 500 IU (in 5dw 50 mL) ivs q 6hr (LDLT POD#9, DDLT POD#7 까지)
16. Tacrolimus (/)mg p.o. bid
17. MMF 750 mg bid
18. Methylprednisolone 60 mg ivs q 24hr
19. HBIG 10,000 IU/20,000 IU + 5%DW 200 mL mivs c 150cc/hr

20. Aspirin coated (Living or split DDLT) : POD #5 start, 100 mg qd
21. SMX-TMP 400 mg/80 mg 1T po.qd (POD #5 start, for 6 months)
22. Esomeprazole 20 mg qd
23. Itraconazole capsule 100 mg bid
24. If HbsAg (+) ⇨ antiviral agent(이전 복용대로 처방)
25. UDCA 200 mg p.o. bid
26. Diomagnite 3.8 g bid
27. Vit. K 10 mg +5DW 50cc miv q 24hr
28. Glutathione 600 mg in NS 50 mL q 12hr
29. L-arginine HCL 15 g +NS 100 mL mivs q 12hr
30. CBC, eletrolyte, chemistry, PT/aPTT/fibrinogen, D-bil, r-GT, LDH, Mg, Ion Ca, S-osm, UA c micro, chest AP (p), USG, CRP, ABGA
31. Gram stain culture & fungus culture: Blood (x2), JP (x3), urine, sputum
32. Tacrolimus level
33. CMV antigenemia (Mon, Wed, Fri)
34. PRN) Pain control; hydromorphone
35. PRN) Quetiapin 25 mg p.o HS for insomnia
36. CBC, PT/aPTT, T-bil/AST/ALT, e'q 12hr
37. Gram stain & culture (C-line tip)

IX. LT POD#6 (GW)

1. V/S q 4hr
2. warming to maintain core temp>36℃
3. Ward ambulation
4. SBD (sterilized porridge)
5. I/O q 8hr (hourly urine check: <1 cc/kg/hr → notify to Dr.)
6. Check Bwt
7. Daily abdominal sterile dressing change
8. BST check q 8hr RI sliding scale

   BST check q 6hrs

   RI sliding MDI

Blood glucose	RI subcut.injection
201 - 250	4
251 - 300	8
301 - 350	12
<80 or > 350	call Dr.

9. 0.1% Chlorohexidine Gargling q 8hr
10. Anti-Thrombin III 500u (in 5dw50 mL) ivs q 6hr
11. Tacrolimus (/)mg po bid--- after confirm
12. MMF 750 mg p.o bid
13. Methylprednisolone 60 mg ivs qd
14. Esomeprazole 20 mg p.o. qd
15. Itraconazole 100 mg p.o. bid
16. If HBsAg (+) ⇨ antiviral agent
17. Diomagnite 3.8 g bid
18. UDCA 200 mg p.o. bid
19. Vit. K 10 mg ivs q qd (until POD#6)
20. Glutathione 600 mg in NS 100 mL q 12hr
21. L-arginine HCL 15 g +NS 100 mL mivs q 12hr

22. HBIG 10,000 IU/20,000 IU + 5%DW 200 mL mivs
23. Aspirin 100 mg p.o. qd (Living or split DDLT)
24. SMX-TMP 1T p.o. qd (for 6 months)
25. CBC, e, chemistry, PT, aPTT, r-GT, D-bil, LDH, Mg, ionized Ca, serum-osm, ammonia, U/A c micro, amLyase, lipase
26. Tacrolimus level
27. CMV antigenemia (Mon, Wed, Fri)
28. Chest AP (p),
29. PRN) Pain control: hydromorphone
30. PRN) Quetiapin 25 mg p.o HS for insomnia

X. LT POD #7

1. V/S q 4hrs in sub ICU
2. Ward ambulation
3. SBD (sterilized porridge)
4. I/O q 8hr (hourly urine check: <1cc/kg/hr → notify to Dr.)
5. Check Body weight
6. Line change: every 4 days
7. Daily abdominal sterile dressing change
8. BST check q 6hrs

   RI sliding MDI

Blood glucose	RI subcut.injection
201 - 250	4
251 - 300	8
301 - 350	12
<80 or > 350	call Dr.

9. 0.1% Chlorohexidine Gargling q 8hr
10. Tacrolimus (/) p.o. bid
11. MMF 750 mg bid
12. Methylprednisolone 60 mg ivs qd
13. Itraconazole 100 mg p.o. bid
14. If HBsAg(+) ⇨ antiviral agent
15. UDCA 200 mg p.o. bid
16. Esomeprazole 20 mg qd
17. Diomagnite 3.8 g bid
18. Glutathione 600 mg in NS 100 mL q 12hr
19. L-arginine HCL 15 g +NS 100 mL mivs q 12hr
20. Aspirin 100 mg p.o. qd (Living or split DDLT)
21. SMX-TMP 1T p.o. qd
22. PRN) hydromorphone 1 mg / 5dw 50cc for pain

23. CBC, e PT/aPTT, chemistry, fibrinogen, D-bil, r-GT, LDH, Mg, Ion Ca, S-osm, ammonia, UA c micro, urine (e, osm), USG, Chest AP (P)

24. Tacrolimus level

25. MPA level (Every Monday and Thursday)

26. CMV antigenemia (Mon, Wed, Fri)

27. AFP, PIVKA-II (only HCC patient)

28. Doppler US F/U

29. PRN) Pain control: hydromorphone

30. PRN) Quetiapin 25 mg p.o HS for insomnia

ABO incompatible Liver Transplantation

I. Adult

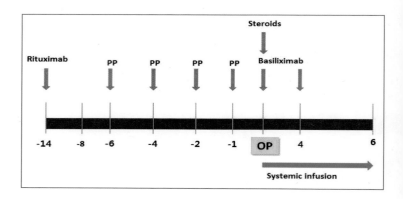

1. Preoperative management

1) Immunosuppression

- Rituximab (375 mg/m²): POD -14 days

- MMF(500mg/bid): Rituximab 주입 다음날부터 복용

2) Plasmapheresis

- POD -6, -4, -2, 1 (if anti-A/B >1:8) - Target: Anti-A/B ≤1:16 ⇨ LT 시행 (LT는 현재 IgM 값 기준)

- Precheck한 isoagglutinin titer에 따라 입원일 결정

- Central line insertion: Access line은 central line으로 16 G이상 (Arrow catheter or I-J catheter)

  Return line은 peripheral line으로 18 G이상 확보, patency 유지

- 진단검사의학과 협진 완료시 스케줄 대로 Plasmapheresis 시행

  : Therapeutic Plasma Exchange, FFP 처방 입력

: Premedication: Chlorpheniramine (Avil) 4 mg 1ⓐ IV, PRN)

- Plasmapheresis 시작 후 매일 isoagglutinin titer 검사 (수술 당일 포함)

- Exchange volume은 기본 1 volume이나 필요시 1.5 volume도 고려

2. Perioperative management

1) Basiliximab induction (20 mg)

2) Systemic infusion (6 days): Steroids, PEG1 & Gabexate mesylate

3. Postoperative management

1) post operative 2~3 weeks : MRCP(MR cholangiopancreaticography (non-contrast)) + Diffusion 촬영

2) Anti-A/B titers - daily check until 2 weeks ⇨ IgM > 1:16, 및 LFT 상승(특히 T.bil) 동반시 적극적으로 plasmapheresis 시행

   - weekly check for first 1 month

   - postoperatively 2, 3, 6 and 12 months

3) 외래에서 plasmapheresis가 고려: Anti-A/B >1:128 (4배 이상 증가시)

Ⅱ. Child

1) Preoperative management - Isoagglutinin titer: 이식 검사시, 입원일, 이식전 7일부터 매일 검사

   - TPE from 7 days before transplantation (-7, -5, -2)

   - Target titer: ≤1:8

2) Intraoperative management

   - 더 많은 Perfusion (3배 이상)

3) Postoperative management

- Isoagglutinin titer: 수술 후 2주까지 매일, 이후 1주에 한번
- 1:64 이상이면 Plasmapheresis

CHAPTER 10.

PEDIATRIC LIVER TRANSPLANTATION

Ⅰ. **Evaluation of Pediatric Liver transplant recipient**

　1) Past medical history

　　(1) Indication of liver transplantation

　　(2) Liver Cirrhosis Complications

　　　① Varix: Endoscopic finding, EVL Hx, bleeding Hx

　　　② Ascites: Ascites control (Diuretics/Tapping), SBP

　　　③ Hepatic Encephalopathy

　　(3) HBV-related: Anti-viral agent, YMDD mutation

　　(4) HCV-related : Anti-viral therapy, HCV Genotype

　　(5) Co-morbid condition

　　　: R/O Hepato-Renal syndrome, R/O Hepato-Pulmonary syndrome

　2) Current status of liver

(1) Liver function test including coagulation profile and platelet count

(2) PELD score

(3) Hepatitis profile

(4) Doppler US

(5) Liver CT

3) R/O Current infection

    (1) History: 최근 1년간 여행력 조사

    (2) Chest PA

      : R/O Pneumonia, R/O Pul. Tbc, R/O Fungal infection

    (3) QuantiFERON-TB

    (4) Viral status

      : anti-HAV (IgG/IgM), automated RPR, anti-HIV, CMV (IgG/IgM), EBV-VCA (IgG/IgM), EBV-EA, EBNA, V-zoster Ab (IgG), HSV2 Ab (IgG), Toxoplasma Ab (IgG/IgM)

    (5) PNS series

    (6) Vaccination history 확인

    (7) Blood culture, Sputum & Urine: Gram stain and culture, Stool culture, Stool exam, Throat, Nasal swab (for MRSA), and Rectal swab (for VRE)

    (8) CRP

    (9) Tumor markers: CEA, AFP

4) Consultation

  : 소아감염, 치과, 이비인후과, 정신과, 사회복지실

5) 간장대기자 등록 서식

간장응급도 1 등록서식

KONOS ID :	(소아)	등록기관명:
대기자명 :		책임자성명:　　　　(인)

정보
- 성 명 : _____ ·생년월일 : ___ 년 ___ 월 ___ 일 · 성별 : □ 남자 □ 여자

- 등록일 : ___ 년 ___ 월 ___ 일　　·관리일자 : ___ 년 ___ 월 ___ 일

임상 정보
- 체중 : ____ kg　·신장 : ____ cm　·혈액형: □ A □ B □ O □ AB　· Rh : □ + □ –

- 진단명 : □ 급성 간부전 □ 윌슨병 □ 기타(_____)

Serology

검사항목	양성	음성	검사항목	양성	음성
HBs Ag			Anti-HCV		
Anti-HBs			Anti-HIV		
Anti-HBc IgM			VDRL		

과거이식여부 : □ 아니오 □ 예 1차 장기명 _____ 이식일자 _____
　　　　　　　　　　　　　　　　2차 장기명 _____ 이식일자 _____

응급도 1 등록 기준
- 18세 미만의 집중치료실에 입원한 급성 또는 만성 간부전증(liver failure)환자가 7일 이내에 간이식을 받지 않으면 생명 연장의 희망이 없는 상태로 다음 중 한가지 이상에 해당하는 경우

① 만성 간질환 없이 간질환의 증상이 나타난 후 8주이내에 뚜렷한 간성혼수가 동반된 급성 전격성 (Fulminant liver failure)환자로, 다음의 3가지 조건중에 한가지 이상을 동반한 경우

　　·인공호흡요법　　·신대체요법　　· INR> 2.0

② 간이식후 7일 이내에 이식된 간이 기능을 하지 못하는 경우(Primary non-function)로 다음 조건 중 2가지 이상을 동반한 경우 (단, 검사결과는 간이식 후 7일 이내 검사결과여야함.)

　　·ALT>=2,000　　·INR>=2.5　　·Total bilirubin >=10mg/dl
　　· 산성혈증(acidosis, 동맥혈 PH<=7.30 혹은 정맥혈 PH<=7.25이거나/혹은Lactate>= 4 mMol/L)

③ 간이식후 14일 이내에 간동맥성 혈전증(hepatic artery thrombosis)이 있는 경우

④ 윌슨병(Wilson's disease) 환자에게 급성 간부전증이 동반된 경우로 ① 항의 조건중 한가지 이상을 동반한 경우
　　　　① 항의 조건 : ·인공호흡요법　　· 신대체요법　　· INR> 2.0

⑤ 만성간질환자중 멜드(펠드)점수가 25점보다 큰 경우(>25)로, 다음 4가지 조건 중 하나를 동반하는 경우
　　·인공호흡요법 유지
　　·소화기계 출혈로 24시간내에 30ml/kg 이상의 적혈구(RBC) 수혈이 필요한 경우
　　·투석이나 CVVH/CVVD가 필요한 신기능장애 혹은 신부전 상태
　　·등록/재등록후 48시간 내에 Glasgow coma scale<10인 경우

6) Pediatric Model for End-Stage Liver Disease : PELD Score

(1) PELD Score

PELD score= $0.436 \times$ (Age)

$- 0.687 \times$ loge Albumin g/dL

$+ 0.480 \times$ loge Bilirubin mg/dL

$+ 1.857 \times$ loge INR

$+ 0.667 \times$ (growth failure)

(Age <1: score 1; Age > 1 : score 0

Growth failure - 2 Standard deviations below mean for age : score

$1 \leq 2$ SD below mean for age: score 0)

Ⅱ. Preparation of Pediatric Liver transplant recipient

1. Transfusion (OR)

(1) Pre-storage leukocyte reduced RBC : 2U (irradiation and filtration)

(2) FFP: 2U

(3) ESP 1U(가능하면) ⇨ ESP 준비 안 되면 LD-PC 2U (irradiation and filtration)

(4) Cryoprecipitate: 2U

2. To OR

(1) Methylprednisolone 20 mg/kg

(2) Hepabig 100 U/kg (30 kg 이상은 10,000 U) : HBV related or Anti-HBc(+) Donor

(3) Antibiotics- Cefotaxime 3 vial, Ampicillin/Sulbactam 1.5 g 6 vial

(4) Albumin 1 bottle

3. To ICU

(1) Dalteparin 1 vial

(2) Gabexate 20 mg/kg

(3) PGE 4 μg/kg

4. Preparation of Intraop. Medication in LT

(1) gabexate (1 vial=100 mg)

- 20 mg/kg mixed in 5DW 24 mL, 1cc/hr

(2) PGE1 (1 amp = 20 mcg)

- 4 μg/kg mixed in 5DW 24 mL, 2cc/hr

(3) dalteparin (1 vial = 10,000 IU/4mL)

- 50 IU/kg mixed in NS 24cc를 만듦. (즉. Bwt> 30 kg이면 0.6 mL), 1cc/hr

- POD#5부터 aspirin start (B.wt < 10 kg이면 25 mg qd)

Ⅲ.Preparation of Pediatric Intestinal Transplant Recipient

1. To OR

(1) Methylprednisolone20 mg/kg

(2) basiliximab

- B.wt ≥ 35 kg ⇨ 20 mg

- B.wt < 35 kg ⇨ 10 mg

(3) Antibiotics- Tazocin + vancomycin

2. To ICU

(1) Fragmin 1 vial

(2) PGE 4 μg/kg

3. Preparation of Intraop. Medication

(1) PGE1 (1 amp = 20 mcg)

- 4 μg/kg mixed in 5DW 24 mL, 2cc/hr

(2) Fragmin (1 vial = 10,000 IU/4 mL)

- 50 IU/kg mixed in NS 24 cc를 만듦. (즉. Bwt > 30 kg이면 0.6 mL), 1cc/hr

- POD#5부터 aspirin start (B.wt < 10 kg이면 25 mg qd)

IMMUNE SUPPRESSION PROTOCOL
A. 면역억제제의 종류와 용법

1. Tacrolimus

1) 투여시작: POD#1 아침부터 시작용량 0.075 mg/kg PO bid

2) 투여 시작 후 약물농도는 반드시 12 ng/mL 정도를 목표로 빨리 올린다 (ITx에서는 15 이상). 이후 trough level은 아래 표를 참고.

3) Target Trough Level of Tacrolimus in LT

OP~1개월	10-12 ng/mL
1개월~3개월	8-10 ng/mL
3개월 이후	5-8 ng/mL

4) Target trough level of tacrolimus in ITx

OP~1개월	15-20 ng/mL
1개월~3개월	12-15 ng/mL
3개월 이후	10-12 ng/mL

2. Steroid

1) Pediatric

(1) Initial at reperfusion; Methylprednisolone 20 mg/kg ivs

(2) POD #1 : Methylprednisolone 10 mg/kg ivs

(3) POD #2 : Methylprednisolone 8 mg/kg ivs

(4) POD #3 : Methylprednisolone 6 mg/kg ivs

(5) POD #4 : Methylprednisolone 4 mg/kg ivs

(6) POD #5 : Methylprednisolone 2 mg/kg ivs

(7) POD #6, #7 : Methylprednisolone 1 mg/kg/day ivs

(8) POD #8~ 1 month Prednisolone (PD) 0.15 mg/kg/day p.o. bid

(9) If rejection (-), tapering & withdrawal around postop 1 month

3. Mycophenolate mofetil

1) 소아에서는 드물게 사용

2) 소아에서 MMF 사용시 용량은 300 mg/m^2 (BSA) PO bid

4. basiliximab (20 mg)

1) 대부분의 소아 LT에서는 사용하지 않는다

2) 학동기 recipient의 경우에는 사용하는 경우가 있기 때문에 confirm 받을 것

3) 소아 ITx와 KT에서는 사용(intraop & POD#4)

4) Usual dose for children and adolescents (aged 1 to 17 years)

① B.wt ≥ 35 kg ⇨ 20 mg

② B.wt < 35 kg ⇨ 10 mg

5. Rituximab

 1) 용량 및 전처치

  (1) 용량: 375 mg/m^2

  (2) PTLD: 2주마다 1번씩 투여하며 총 4번 투여한다.

  (3) 전처치

   ■ Oral acetaminophen 650 mg

   ■ Oral diphenylhydramine 50 mg

B. Immunosuppression Protocol for Pediatric transplantation recipient

1. Liver transplantation

 1) basiliximab 사용하지 않는다.

 2) MMF 사용 안 함.

 3) tacrolimus과 steroid의 이중요법을 사용

  (1) 따라서 tacrolimus를 POD 1 day부터 oral로 사용하며 level을 특히 strict하게 유지한다.

2. Intestinal transplantation

 1) basiliximab로 induction 한다.

 2) tacrolimus과 steroid의 이중요법을 사용: 따라서 tacrolimus를 POD 1 day부터 oral로 사용하며 level을 높게 유지한다.

3. Kidney transplantation

 1) Induction with basiliximab (Preop. & POD #4) + tacrolimus (0.075 mg/kg/dose bid)+MMF (300 mg/m^2/dose bid)+steroid

 2) Steroid tapering starting at 1 wk, withdrawal in 1 month

3) basiliximab : ≥ 35 kg ➪ 20 mg, < 35 kg ➪ 10 mg 사용한다.

4) MMF 용량은 300 mg/m² (BSA) PO bid

C. Treatment for Acute Rejection

1. Steroid (SPT, Steroid pulse therapy)

1) Schedule

(1) Children < 40 kg

- Bolus (3days) 10 mg/kg IV, and then tapering (daily half dose)

- Resume oral PD at maintenance (0.15 mg/kg po bid)

(2) If B.wt ≥ 40 kg

- Adult dosage 적용

(3) Ganciclovir start (prophylactic dose): resume PO acyclovir with po PD

(4) Anti-ulcer medication (Intravenous H2 blocker)

(5) CNI level: 점차 올려 SPT 끝날 때 10 ng/mL로 유지

(6) CMV antigenemia check 월,수,금

INFECTION IN TRANSPLANT RECIPIENTS

A. Pre-Transplant Evaluation for infectious disease

1. Donor evaluation

1) Deceased Donor

(1) Serology: HBsAg, anti-HBs, anti-HBc (IgG), anti-HCV, anti-HAV (IgG), VDRL (automated RPR), anti-HIV, CMV (IgG), EBV-VCA (IgG)

(2) Culture: Blood, Urine, Sputum Gram stain & culture (including

fungus)

2) Living Donor

: HBsAg, anti-HBs, anti-HBc (IgG), anti-HCV, anti-HAV (IgG), VDRL (automated RPR), anti-HIV, CMV (IgG), EBV-VCA (IgG)

2. Recipient evaluation

1) HBV : HBsAg, anti-HBs, anti-HBc (IgG), HBeAg, anti-HBe, HBV DNA Quantitation, HBV YMDD mutation

2) HCV : anti-HCV (IgG), HCV RNA detection or HCV RNA Quantitation, HCV genotype

3) anti-HAV (IgG/IgM), VDRL (automated RPR), anti-HIV,

4) CMV (IgG/IgM), EBV-VCA (IgG/IgM), EBV-EA, EBNA, V-zoster Ab (IgG), HSV2 Ab (IgG), Toxoplasma Ab (IgG/IgM),

5) Blood Culture 3회

6) Gram stain & culture (include fungus)- Urine, Throat, Sputum & Stool, Nasal swab (for MRSA), Rectal Swab (for VRE)

7) Stool exam

8) QunatiFERON-TB

9) Vaccination - Influenza, Pneumococcal, Tetanus

B. Post-Transplant management of infection

1. Postoperative Routine Surveillance

1) Ordinary Bacteria and Fungus

(1) Urine, Sputum (or Throat), Drains, Bile, Wounds, Blood culture for bacteria and fungus ⇨ daily

(2) While hospitalized after then --> if (+), consult Division of

Infectious Diseases

(3) infection의 증거나, FUO 등이 있으면 수시로 F/U culture를 한다.

(4) culture결과가 나오면 담당 fellow와 상의해서 항생제의 추가나 change를 고려하고 감염내과에 consult도 고려한다.

2) CMV

(1) CMV antigenemia surveillance

① Immediate Post-Op recipient, high-risk recipients, antigenemia positive recipients or CMV disease recipients

: frequently f/u한다(월, 수, 금 - 이식 후 1주일 동안).

② weekly while hospitalized(매주 월요일)

③ After discharge, at every visit (q 4 weeks) till post-op. 12 months

④ In case of fever or leukopenia of unknown cause

⑤ CMV infection 없이 f/u 검사

   i) 이식 후 첫 1주는 월, 수, 금 검사

   ii) 이식 후 1달까지는 매주 시행

   iii) 1달 이후부터는 이식 후 1년까지는 1달에 1번 검사한다.

⑥ CMV infection으로 ganciclovir 투여 중인 경우(preemptive treatment시) 또는 Steroid pulse therapy시 월,수,금 검사한다.

(2) CMV PCR

3) EBV

(1) EBV-VCA (IgG/IgM), EBV-EA, EBNA

: less reliable for post-transplant surveillance

(2) EBV Quantitative PCR

① High-risk patients

   i) Transplant from EBV Ig G (+) donor to EBV Ig G (-) recipient

      ii) All children < 1 yr regardless of pretransplant serology

    ② PreOp ~ PostOp 1 yr - every 1 month

      ~ PostOp 2 yr - q 2 months

      이후 - q 4 months

4) HBV: Hepatitis profile, HBV DNA Quantitation

5) HCV: HCV RNA Detection

6) HCV RNA Quantitation

7) HHV-6 detection PCR

2. Prevention and treatment of infection

1) Bacterial and protozoal infections

  가. Bacterial prophylaxis

  (1) Systemic antibiotics

    ① LT

     : Cefotaxime 30-40 mg/kg IV q 8hr (AST) and Ampicillin-sulbactam 50 mg/kg IV q 6hr (AST)

    ② ITx

     : Tazocin 100 mg/kg q 6 hrs

    ③ KT

     : Ceftizoxime 1.0 mg iv q 12hr

    ④ Start with induction

    ⑤ Reinjection intraoperatively in case of prolonged surgery

    ⑥ Duration: POD#2까지

    ⑦ Sepsis등으로 수술 전에 쓰던 항생제가 있다면 지속한다

  (2) Selective Bowel Decontamination

    시행하지 않는다.

(3) Prophylactic antibiotics during procedures

① Cefotaxime and ubacillin with invasive procedures (for 2~3 days)

② Cholangiography, PTBD, ERBD, ENBD, angiography, balloon dilatation, stent insertion, biopsy, PCD, etc.

2) Pneumocystis infection prophylaxis (Pneumocystis jiroveci)

(1) SMX-TMP (Sulfamethoxazole/Trimethoprim) (syrup or tab) 750 mg/m^2/day를 2회로 나누어 줌 cf)본원 SMX-TMP syrup은 1 mL 중 TMP 8 mb,SUL 40 mg, SMX-TMP tablet은 TMP 80 mg/SUL 400 mg임

(2) Start at the beginning of oral intake. 매주 토요일, 일요일(6개월간)

3) Prevention for Fungal infection

(1) Itraconazole syrup 2.5 mg/kg bid (during NPO)

(2) Diet시작 후부터 itraconazole 2.5 mg/kg bid (till POD#30)

(3) ITx: Fluconazole IV 5 mg/kg q 24hrs (for 2 weeks)

4) Viral infection

(1) CMV

① Prophylaxis

i) CMV Donor IgG (+) / Recipient IgG (-) : IV ganciclovir prophylaxis for 2 weeks ⇨ no further prophylactic antiviral Tx

ii) during SPT: IV ganciclovir prophylaxis

② CMV prophylaxis in ITx

i) High risk (D+/R- or r-ATG induction)

(i) IV ganciclovir 2.5 mg/kg q 12 hrs for 2 weeks

(ii) Cytogam

       A. POD#3 150 mg/kg

       B. POD#17 100 mg/kg q 1 week x 4 doses

    (iii) Valgancyclovir 14 mg/kg qd for 6 months

  ii) Intermediate risk (D+/R+ or D-/R+)

    (i)   IV ganciclovir 2.5 mg/kg q 12 hrs for 2 weeks

    (ii) Valgancyclovir 14 mg/kg qd for 3 months

  iii) Low risk (D-/R-)

    (i)   IV ganciclovir 2.5 mg/kg q 12 hrs for 2 weeks

    (ii) Acyclovir 20 mg/kg pot id for 3 months

③ CMV antigenemia

  i)   이식 후 1달 이내: 매주 월요일마다 검사한다.

     → 만약 CMV antigenemia가 양성이면 월, 수, 금 검사한다.

  ii) 이식 후 1달이 지나면 매달 1번씩 검사한다.

④ Preemptive therapy

  i)   If CMV antigenemia > 10/400,000

  ii) Ganciclovir (IV) until CMV antigenemia is negative (minimum 7 days)

  iii) 소아 KT에서는 CMV high risk 환아를 제외한 환자들은 valacyclovir를 복용하지 않는다.

⑤ Treatment of established CMV disease

  i)   Ganciclovir (IV) for 2~4 wks

  ii) F/U CMV disease: EGD, Sigmoidoscopy or colonoscopy, Biopsy

  iii) Other agents: ganciclovir-resistant CMV → Foscarnet

Ganciclovir (DHPG)				
	Treatment dose		Prophylactic dose	
CCr	Dose	Dosing Interval	Dose	Dosing Interval
(mL/min)	(mg/kg)	(hrs)	(mg/kg)	(hrs)
>70	5.0	12	5.0	24
50-69	2.5	12	2.5	24
25-49	2.5	24	1.25	24
10-24	1.25	24	0.625	24
<10	1.25	투석 후 주3회	0.625	투석 후 주3회

iv) If granulocyte $<$ 1,000/mm^3 or platelet $<$ 20,000/mm^3 : discontinue ganciclovir

(2) EBV

Am J Transplant 2004;4(S10):59

① Prophylaxis

   i) Ganciclovir (IV) for POD 2 wks and then acyclovir (PO) for 2 years

   ii) High-risk patients

      (i) Transplant from EBV IgG (+) donor to EBV IgG (-) recipient

      (ii) All children $<$ 1 yr regardless of pretransplant serology

② Acyclovir Dose (04. 4. 6 이후)

   i) 2세 이상 – 200 mg q 4 hr (5회)

   ii) 2세 이하 – 100 mg q 4 hr (5회)

③ PTLD (posttransplant lymphoproliferative disease)

   i) Risk factors of PTLD

      (i) ATG와 같은 면역억제제 사용자

(ii) EBV D+/R- status

(iii) Fewer HLA matching

(iv) CMV D+/R- and CMV disease

(v) 이러한 risk factor가 있는 환자에서 fever, lymphadeno-pathy, diarrhea, allograft dysfunction 등의 증상이 있으면 PTLD에 대한 aggressive work up

ii) PTLD의 진단 및 management

    (i) P/E for cervical/axillary/inguinal LN enlargement

    (ii) Abdomen US or CT for detection of LN enlargement

    (iii) Mucosa biopsy via sigmoidoscopy (colonoscopy)

    (iv) LN biopsy, if palpable or enlarged

    (v) Tonsillectomy (biopsy)

    (vi) reduction of immunosuppression

- ◆ ↓ cyclosporine/tacrolimus to $\frac{1}{2}$ or less
- ◆ Stop azathioprine/MMF
- ◆ Maintain oral steroid
- ◆ Time to response; 2-4 wks

    (vii) Anti-CD20 antibodies (Rituximab − 375 mg/m^2)

- ◆ Neutralizing the B-cells expressing CD20
- ◆ Abort the lytic-replicative phase of EBV-driven lymphoproliferation

iii) A high EBV DNA load (EBV PCR > 2000 copies/5 μL whole blood) in the peripheral blood has been associated with an increased risk on PTLD.

   (i)   Reduction of immunosuppression

   (ii) Antiviral medication ± IVIG

   (iii) Monoclonal B-cell antibody therapy

   (iv) Surgical resection

   iv) Baseline study in pediatric LT : EBV (3)

Preop~Postop 1yr	Every 1 month
~Postop 2yr	q 2 months
~이후	q 4 months

(3) VZV, HSV

① No prophylaxis

② Treatment for Herpes infection

   : Acyclovir 10-14 days

③ Dose of Intravenous Acyclovir

CCr (mL/min)	Induction Dose (mg/kg)	Dosing Interval (hrs)
>50	10	8
25-50	10	12
10-24	10	24
<10	5	24

④ Dose of Oral Acyclovir

CCr (mL/min)	Induction Dose (mg/kg)	Dosing Interval (hrs)
>50	800mg	6
10-50	800mg	8
<10	800mg	24

(4) HBV infection in LT

① De novo hepatitis B prophylaxis in HBcAb (+) donor

    i)   Hepabig 100 U/kg ivs + 5%DW 100cc mix IV

    ii)   intraop시 anhepatic phase에 주고, 수술 후 6일째까지 총 7번을 준다.

    iii)   이후 HBs-Ab titer > 200 되도록 HBIG 2,000 U IV

    iv)   소아의 경우 POD 1 yr 후 active vaccination (Hepavax, Euvax)으로 전환(HBs-Ab titer 100이상 유지)

② HBcAb (+) group이 아닌 소아환자(HBsAg (-) 환아 포함)

  : Hepatitis profile 6개월마다 f/u and HBs-Ab titer 10이상 유지

(5) Tuberculosis Prophylaxis

① 전염성 결핵 환자와 최근 접촉이 있었던 환자

② Chest PA에서 stable Tb. 병변이 있으면서 이전에 결핵 치료력이 없거나 부적절하게 치료를 받았다고 여겨지는 환자에서 QuantiFERON 양성 환자

③ Regimen: INH 300 mg(9개월) + B6 50 mg

POST-TRANSPLANT MANAGEMENT

A. Post-operative management of Liver Transplantation

  1. POD#3부터 oral intake 진행(SOW ⇨ SBD or formula feeding)

  2. Post-Op Studies

    1) Doppler USG : POD#1, 3, (5), 7, 14

    2) DISIDA: POD#14

    3) chest X-ray는 ICU에 있는 동안에는 daily check하고, L-tube나

drain 등의 위치 확인을 위해서 simple abdomen도 가능한 확인을
한다.

4) 소아에서는 CT는 가능한 시행하지 않는다.

3. 식이 시작시부터 ambroxol, pantoprazole, diogel, UDCA
PO medi start

1) UDCA 용량

(1) < 10 kg	50 mg bid
(2) 10~20 kg	100 mg bid
(3) > 20 kg	100 mg tid

4. POD#5부터 aspirin overlap (aspirin micro)

1) < 10 kg	25 mg qd
2) 10~20 kg	50 mg qd
3) > 20 kg	100 mg qd

B. Post-operative management of Intestinal transplantation

1. POD#5~6에 tolerable하면 L-tube clamping(2시간 clamp/2시간 declamp) 시도

2. POD#6~7에 tolerable하면 L-tube 24hr clamping

3. POD#7에 initial ileoscopy & Bx ⇨ 정상소견이면 enteral feeding 시작 고려

4. Initial EN: Vivonex-TEN 1/2 strength 5 cc/hr continuous feeding start

5. EN feeding 증량은 환자가 tolerable한 범위 내에서 진행, 2/3 strength Vivonex-TEN으로 full EN을 목표로 함

6. Vivonex-TEN 1 month, Neocate Jr 1 month, 이후 Nutren Jr 순서로 진행

7. Oral feeding은 소량씩, as tolerated

8. Stool output은 45~50 cc/kg/day까지 tolerable, 35 cc/kg/day 부터는 초과량을 1/2NS로 replace

C. Out-Patient follow up

1. Pediatric LT

1) Doppler: 3개월마다 F/U(3년까지), 1년 마다 F/U(3년이후)

2) CT: 3년마다 F/U check

3) CMV antigenemia: routine(매달)

4) Steroid tapering and withdrawal (Post-Op. 3 months)

5) 대부분의 drug은 6개월까지

6) UDCA 용량

    (1) < 10 kg   50 mg bid

    (2) 10~20 kg   100 mg bid

    (3) > 20 kg   100 mg tid

7) EBV-high risk recipient

    (1) EBV Quantitative PCR: 매 외래 내원 시(매달)

    (2) Serology: EB-VCA (IgG/M), EBV-EA, EBNA(6개월마다) EBV (IgG) positive conversion 시 더 이상 시행 안 함.

    (3) A high EBV DNA load (EBV PCR > 2000 copies/5 μL whole blood) in the peripheral blood is associated with an increased risk on PTLD

8) autoimmune Ab.(IgG, FANA,SMA,ANA) 검사를 연 1회 시행한다.

9) LT후 퇴원 전 PS 협진하여 적절한 wound care 받도록 한다.

10) Vaccination

	처방	비고
Influenza	1 vial IM(성인)	매년
Hepatitis A	1 vial IM (성인, 16세 이상)	HAV IgG 음성인 경우
Pneumococcal vaccine (polysaccharide vaccine)	1 vial IM	- 이식 전 검사 시 1회 접종 - 이식 후 5년 지나서 추가 접종을 1회 더 한다.
Tetanus (Td)	1 vial IM	- 40세 이상: 3회 (0, 1-2m, 6-12m) , 이후에는 10년마다 1회 - 40세 미만: 10년마다 1회

Pediatric Liver Transplantation

I. PreOp. Order (POD# -1)

1. V/S q 8 hr
2. W/A
3. NPO
4. Check B. Wt.
5. Get Op Permission
6. L-tube prep
7. Go to OR with chart
8. Antiembolic cuff to OR
9. Anti-embolic cuff preparation
10. Antibiotics skin test: Ampicillin/sulbactam, cefotaxime
11. NS 1L iv 60 cc/hr
12. Famotidine 0.5A + NS 50 mL mivs at 6am
13. alprostadil 4 μg/kg (in 5DW 24 mL x2) prep to ICU
    5DW 50cc
14. gabexate 20 mg/kg (in 5DW 24 mL)   prep to ICU
15. Fragmin 50 μ/kg (in N/S 24 mL)   prep to ICU
16. Solumedrol 20 mg/kg   prep to OR
17. Hepabig 100 unit/kg (Donor: anti-HBc (+)) prep to OR
18. 5% albumin 1 bottle   prep to OR
19. Ampicillin/sulbactam 50 mg/kg iv q 8hrs
20. Cefotaxime 30~40 mg/kg iv q 8hrs
21. CBC with Diff., Chemistry profile, Electrolyte, Ammonia, TCO2, Amylase/Lipase, PT/aPTT, CRP, fibrinogen
22. HLA crossmatch, HLA-A, B typing (DNA), HLA-DR Typing (DNA) (기존 검사결과있으면 안해도 됨)
23. Blood culture *3 with fungus culture
24. Gram stain and Culture (Urine, Sputum, stool, throat swab),

25. Fungus culture (Urine, Sputum, stool, throat swab)
26. Gram stain and Culture: Nasal swab –MRSA, Rectal swab-VRE
27. Antithrombin III activity
28. EBV-PCR quan

Ⅱ. POSTOP. ORDER

1. V/S q 15 min until stable, then q 30 minX4, then q 1 hr

   : warming to maintain core temp >36'C

2. BR

3. NPO

4. I/O q 8 hr (hourly urine check < 1 cc/kg/hr -> noti)

5. CVP monitoring q 1hr

   If > 8 mmHg or < 3 mmHg -----Notify to Dr

6. Keep A-Line with continuous monItoring

   If BP > 130/100 mmHg or < 90/50 mmHg ---- Notify to Dr.

7. Check Bwt & A/C

8. Keep Foley in situ

9. JP drains to closed drainage

10. L-tube aspiration q 4 hr

11. Position change q 2 hr

12. E-tube suction q 4 hr & postural drainage q 4 hr

13. Ventilator Care

   - HOB 30도

   - DVT prophylaxis IPC

   - Stress ulcer drug prophylaxis

   - Pain assess q 8hrs

   - Sedation scale q 8hrs

   - RASS+1 이상일 때 억제대 적용

14. BST check q 6 hr

   : If BGL <140 or >240, △BGL >120 ⇨ recheck 2hrs later

      1) **Initiation**

         (1) 180 mg/dl < BGL < 240 mg/dl ⇨ starting rate: 1unit/hr

         (2) 240 mg/dl < BGL ⇨ starting rate: 2unit/hr

      2) ** Maintenance**

(1) BGL < 100 ⇨ stop for 2hrs & notify & restart when >180 by rate -1unit/hr

(2) 100 < BGL < 140 ⇨ rate -1units/hr

(3) 140 < BGL < 180 ⇨ maintain rate

(4) 180 < BGL < 240 ⇨ rate +1unit/hr (maintain if BGL is decreasing)

(5) 240 < BGL < 300 ⇨ rate +2unit/hr (maintain if BGL is decreasing)

(6) 300< BGL ⇨ rate +2unit/hr & notify

15. 12 hr urine collection for Ccr

16. 0.12% Chlorhexidine gargling q 6 hr

17. 10% Dextrose 500 mL miv c 30cc/hr

    2M NaCl 20mEq

    Tamipool 1/2 A

18. alprostadil 4 mcg/kg (in 5DW 24 mL) x2 mivs c 2 cc/hr

19. gabexate 20 mg/kg (in 5DW 24 mL) mivs c 1 cc/hr

20. Fragmin 50 u/kg (in N/S 24 mL) mivs c 1cc/hr

21. Anti-Thrombin III 100 u (in N/S/10mL) ivs q 6hr

22. Cefotaxim30~40 mg/kg (in N/S 5 mL) ivs q 8hr

23. Ampicillin-sulbactam 50 mg/kg (in N/S 5 mL) ivs q 8hr

24. Ganciclovir 5 mg/kg ivs (CMV prophylaxis or EBV high risk group)

25. Itraconazole syrup p.o. bid (2.5 mg/kg)

26. Ambroxol 1/4A ivs q 12 hr

27. Famotidine 1/4 A(in N/S 5 mL) mivs q 12 hr

28. Vt. K 1/4 A ivs qD

29. Diogel 1/4P plt q 6 hr

30. Chest AP (p)

31. CBC with diff. Count q 6 hr

32. PT/aPTT, electrolyte, BUN/Cr, Albumin, T. Bil, GOT/GPT, ABGA q 6 hr

33. Chemistry profile, D-Bil, , r-GTP, LDH, Ammonia, Mg, ionized Ca, S-Osm, CRP

34. Fibrinogen, FDP q 12hr

35. Anti-Thrombin III

36. U/A c micro. Urine E'/Osm

Ⅲ. Pediatric LT POD #1

1. V/S q 1 hr
   : warming to maintain core temp >36'C
2. BR
3. NPO
4. I/O q 8 hr (houry urine check < 1 cc/kg/hr -> noti)
5. CVP monltoring q 1hr
   If > 8 mmHg or < 3 mmHg -----Notify to Dr
6. Keep A-Line with continuous monltoring
   If BP > 130/100 mmHg or < 90/50 mmHg ---- Notify to Dr.
7. Check Bwt & A/C
8. Keep Foley in situ
9. JP drains to closed drainage
10. L-tube aspiration q 4 hr
11. E-tube suction q 4 hr & postural drainage q 4 hr
12. Ventilator Care
    HOB 30도
    DVT prophylaxis IPC
    Stress ulcer drug prophylaxis
    Pain assess q 8hrs
    Sedation scale q 8hrs
    RASS+1 이상일 때 억제대 적용
13. Line change : every 4 days
14. Daily abdominal sterile dressing change
15. BST chesk q 6 hr
    : If BGL <140 or >240, △BGL >120 ⇨ recheck 2hrs later
    1) **Initiation**
       (1) 180 mg/dl < BGL < 240 mg/dl ⇨ starting rate: 1unit/hr
       (2) 240 mg/dl < BGL ⇨ starting rate: 2unit/hr
    2) **Maintenance**
       (1) BGL < 100 ⇨ stop for 2hrs & notify & restart when >180 by rate -1unit/hr
       (2) 100 < BGL < 140 ⇨ rate -2units/hr
       (3) 140 < BGL < 180 ⇨ maintain rate
       (4) 180 < BGL < 240 ⇨ rate +1unit/hr(감소 추세일 경우 maintain)
       (5) 240 < BGL < 300 ⇨ rate +2unit/hr(감소 추세일 경우 maintain)
       (6) 300 < BGL ⇨ rate +2unit/hr & notify
16. 0.1 % chlorhexidine gargling q 8 hr
17. 10% Dextrose 500 mL miv c 30

cc/hr

2M NaCl 30mEq

2M KCl 10mEq

Tamipool 1/2 A

18. alprostadil 4 mcg/kg (in 5DW 24 mL) x2 mivs c 2 cc/hr

19. gabexate 20 mg/kg (in 5DW 24 mL) mivs c 1 cc/hr

20. Fragmin 50 u/kg (in N/S 24 mL) mivs c 1 cc/hr

21. Anti-Thrombin III 100u (in N/S/10 mL) ivs q 6hr

22. FK ( ) mg PLT bid (POD#1 start)

23. Methyprednisolone 10 mg/kg ivs q D

24. Cefotaxim30~40 mg/kg (in N/S 5 mL) ivs q 8hr

25. Ampicillin/sulbactam 50 mg/kg (in N/S 5 mL) ivs q 8hr

26. Ganciclovir 5 mg/kg ivs (CMV prophylaxis or EBV high risk group) according to CCr

- CMV IgG (-) recipient from CMV IgG (+) Donor : 2주간 Ganciclovir IV

- EBV high risk group

: 2주간 Ganciclovir IV

2주 이후 2년간 Acyclovir 100 mg(2세이하) q 4hr(5회/day)

Acyclovir 200 mg(2세이상) q 4hr(5회/day)

27. Hepabig 100unit/kg (in 5DW 20 mL) mivs over 4 hr (Avil 1/4A ivs) (anti-HBc (+) group)

28. Itraconazole syrup p.o. bid (2.5 mg/kg)

29. Ambroxol 1/4A ivs q 12 hr

30. Famotidine 1/4 A (in N/S 5 mL) mivs q 12 hr

31. Vt. K 1/4 A ivs qd

32. Diogel 1/4P plt q 6 hr

33. Infantogram (p)

34. CBC with diff. Count q 8 hr

35. PT/aPTT, electrolyte, BUN/Cr, Albumin, T. Bil, GOT/GPT, ABGA q 8 hr

36. Chemistry profile, D-Bil, r-GTP, LDH, Ammonia, Mg, ionized Ca, S-Osm, CRP

37. Fibrinogen, FDP qd

38. Anti-Thrombin III

39. U/A c micro. Urine E'/Osm

40. Gram stain & Culture and Fungus Culture, Urine, Sputum, Blood (X1), JP (X2)

41. CMV antigenemia(월, 수, 금)

42. Doppler US: Consultation

Ⅳ. Pediatric LT POD #2

1. V/S q 1 hr
   : warming to maintain core temp >36'C
2. BR
3. NPO
4. I/O q 8 hr(hourly urine check <1cc/kg/hr -> noti)
5. CVP monitoring q 1hr
   If > 8 cmH$_2$O or < 3 cmH$_2$O -----Notify to Dr
6. Keep A-Line with continuous monltoring
   If BP > 130/100 mmHg or < 90/50 mmHg ---- Notify to Dr.
7. Check Bwt & A/C
8. Keep Foley in situ
9. JP drains to closed drainage
10. L-tube aspiration q 4 hr
11. Position change q 2 hr
12. E-tube suction q 4 hr & postural drainage q 4 hr
13. Line change : every 4 days
14. Daily abdominal sterile dressing change
15. BST check q 6 hr
    : If BGL <140 or >240, △BGL >120 ⇨ recheck 2hrs later
    1) ** Initiation**
       (1) 180 mg/dl< BGL < 240 mg/dl ⇨ starting rate: 1unit/hr
       (2) 240 mg/dl < BGL ⇨ starting rate: 2unit/hr
    2) ** Maintenance**
       Maintenance
       (1) BGL < 100 ⇨ stop for 2hrs & notify & restart when >180 by rate -1unit/hr
       (2) 100 < BGL < 140 ⇨ rate -2units/hr
       (3) 140 < BGL < 180 ⇨ maintain rate
       (4) 180 < BGL < 240 ⇨ rate +1unit/hr(감소 추세일 경우 maintain)
       (5) 240 < BGL < 300 ⇨ rate +2unit/hr(감소 추세일 경우 maintain)
       (6) 300 < BGL ⇨ rate +2unit/hr & notify
16. 0.1 % Hibitane gargling q 8 hr
17. 10% Dextrose 500 mL miv c 30 cc/hr
    2M NaCl 30mEq

2M KCl 10 mEq

Tamipool 1/2 A

18. alprostadil 4ug/kg (in 5DW 24 mL) x2 mivs c 2cc/hr
    : POD#3에 1/3로 감량하여 POD#6까지

19. 20 mg/kg (in 5DW 24 mL) mivs c 1 cc/hr

20. Fragmin 50 u/kg (in N/S 24 mL) mivs c 1 cc/hr

21. Anti-Thrombin III 100u(in N/S/10mL) ivs q 6hr

22. tacrolimus ( ) mg bid

23. Methylprednisolone 8 mg/kg ivs q D

24. Cefotaxim 30~40 mg/kg (in N/S 5 mL) ivs q 8hr

25. Ubacillin 50 mg/kg (in N/S 5 mL) ivs q 8hr

26. Ganciclovir 5 mg/kg ivs (EBV high risk group) : adjustment according to Ccr

27. Hepabig 100 U/kg (in N/S 20 mL) mivs over 4 hr (Avil 1/4A ivs)(HBc (+) group)

28. Itraconazole syrup p.o. bid (2.5 mg/kg)

29. Ambroxol 1/4A ivs q 12 hr

30. Famotidine 1/4 A (in N/S 5 mL) mivs q 12 hr

31. Vt. K 1/4 A ivs qD

32. Diogel 1/4P plt q 6 hr

33. Infantogram (p)

34. CBC with diff. Count q 8 hr

35. PT/aPTT,, electrolyte, BUN/Cr, Albumin, T. Bil, GOT/GPT, ABGA q 8 hr

36. Chemistry profile, D-Bil, , r-GTP, LDH, Ammonia, Mg, ionized Ca, S-Osm

37. Fibrinogen, FDP

38. Anti-Thrombin III

39. U/A c micro. Urine E'/Osm

40. Gram stain & Culture and Fungus culture, Urine, Sputum, Blood (X1), JP (X2)

41. tacrolimus level

42. CMV antigenemia(월, 수, 금)

43. Doppler US : Consultation (POD#3)

V. Pediatric LT POD #3 이후

1. POD#3~4부터 식이 진행
2. 식이 시작 시부터 ambroxol, pantoprazole, diogel, UDCA PO medi start
3. POD#5부터 aspirin overlap (aspirin micro)
   - ◆ < 10 kg   25 mg qd
   - ◆ 10~20 kg   50 mg qd
   - ◆ > 20 kg 100 mg qd
4. UDCA 용량
   - ◆ < 10 Kg   50 mg bid
   - ◆ 10~20 kg   100 mg bid
   - ◆ 20 kg   100 mg tid

CHAPTER 11.

KT RECIPIENT EVALUATION

I. General concept

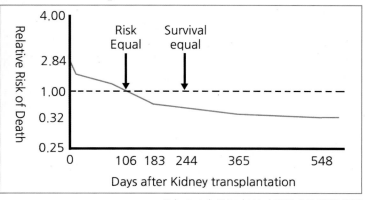

Robert et al., N Engl J Med 1999; 341:1725-1730

☞ The relative risk of death among transplant recipients, as compared with patients on the waiting list, adjusted for other factors.

II. Evaluation of recipient organ state

1. Past medical history

1) Cause of renal failure

: Chronic GN, IgA nephropathy, DM nephropathy, HTN nephropathy, PCKD

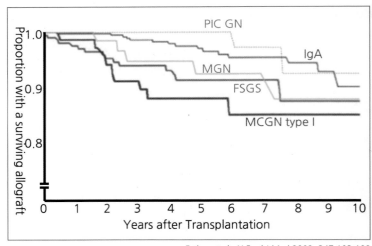

Esther et al., N Engl J Med 2002; 347:103-109

☞ Allograft loss due to recurrence of GN was different according to the type of GN.

* Nephrectomy of native kidney in PCKD pateints.

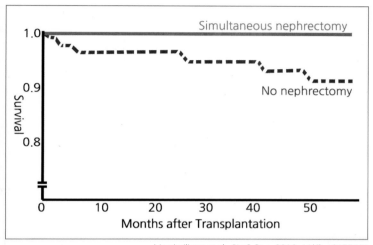

Massimiliano et al., PLoS One. 2016; 11(6): e0155481

☞ Simultaneous ipsilateral nephrectomy for PCKD patients did better effect.

Indication : hematuria, infection, small space for KT due to large PCKD, etc.

2) Dialysis modality : HD or PD, patency of vascular access

3) Daily Urine volume

4) Previous KT history

5) Co-morbid disease and current medication

: DM, Hypertension, HBV/HCV status

III. Evaluation of recipient organ state

1. Voiding cystourethrography (VCUG)

1) Vesicoureteral reflux (VUR)

   : High-grade VUR is accompanied by a higher risk of UTI, even if it was not a problem before KT. In that case, nephrectomy can be the surgical option

   (Erturk et al., Urology 1998 May;51:27-30).

2) Bladder capacity

   : Estimated bladder capacity in ESRD patients = Bwt (Kg) × 7 mL

   (Kidney transplantation 7th p.177)

3) Check other urologic intervention or operation history.

2. Abdomen CT

1) Check vascular anatomy.

2) Ipsilateral nephrectomy also needed when the large PCKD cover the available space for KT.

3. Duplex US of lower extremity

: for check of iliac artery calcification or stenosis.

IV. R/O Current infection

1. History : recent travel history

2. Viral status : HBs Ag/Anti-HBs Antibody/HBcAb (IgG), HAVAb (IgG), Anti-HCV Antibody, Anti-HIV Antibody, automated RPR, anti-HIV, CMV (IgG), EBV-VCA (IgG), HSV2 Ab (IgG), EBNA , EBV -EA, VZV Antibody (IgG), Toxoplasma Antibody (IgG), HSV (1+2) Antibody IgG,

Polyomavirus (2 days prior to KT), Parvovirus (2 days prior to KT)

3. Chest PA/Chest CT : check Pneumonia, Pulmonary Tuberculosis, Fungal infection

4. QuantiFERON-TB

5. PNS series/OMU CT

6. Confirm vaccination – Pneumococcal, Influenza

7. Blood culture, Sputum & Urine: Gram stain and culture, Stool culture, Stool exam

   Throat, Nasal swab (for MRSA), and Rectal swab (for VRE)

V. Routine Lab

1. ABO/Rh typing &Ab screen (T&S), Isoagglutinin Titer (in case of ABOi KT)

2. HLA A/B/DR/DQ Typing (DNA)

3. HLA crossmatch (CDC), HLA Crossmatch, Flow Cytometry

4. HLA Ab Single Identification, Class I/II

5. Mammography (married female), Breast US (unmarried female), Bone densitometry, EGD, colonoscopy (over 50 year old), VCUG Sonography : LGP, Adrenal, Kidney & Bladder Abdomen & pevic CT, CT angiography (intracranial arteries) (in PCKD case)

VI. HLA crossmatch

1. CDC, T & B cell- Flow cytometry ⇨ 1 days prior to KT

   1) HLA Ab Single Identification, Class I/II ⇨ if there is no result within 3 months.

2) In the case of desensitization, check CDC, Flow cytometry just before KT.

VII. Cardiovascular evaluation

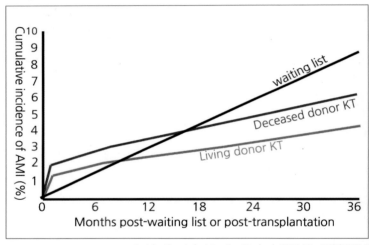

Kasiske BL, et al., J Am Soc Nephrol. 2006 Mar;17(3):900-7

☞ The risk of Myocaridal Infarction is increasing in ESRD patients regardless KT status.

1) ECG Routine, Advanced Echocardiography

2) In case of Asymptomatic, DM (+) & Age>60, CABG or PCI history (+)

: Carotid duplex US, Lower extremity duplex US, pre-stress Echocardiography

3) In case of Symptomatic, DM (+) & Age>60, CABG or PCI history (+)

: Exercise stress Echocardiography

VIII. Consultation

: Dental, ENT, OBGY, infectionist, Social service

Psychiatric, if necessary

IX. KT recipient check criteria

Routine Lab	If admitted to hospital recheck	
Viral maker		
Chest x-ray EKG Routine PFT (spirometry and F/V curve) Advanced echo		
Duplex US, Carotid & Lower extremity	if there is no result within 6mo	
Liver, GB & Pancreas US	if there is no result within 1year	If abnormal, proceed with careful consideration
VCUG	if there is no result	
Esophagogastroduodenoscopy	if there is no result within 1year	
Colonoscopy	if there is no result within 3year (if age > 50y)	

** Patients with type I DM who are hospitalized for LDKT and DDKT should be considered whether the patients need pancreas after kidney transplant (PAK) and should proceed to the left incision at the time of KT.

X. Admission schedule according to the ABO isoagg-lutinin titer

1) ≤ 1: 32   → 7 days ago

2) 1: 64 ~ 1: 128   → 10 days ago

3) ≥ 1: 256   → 2 weeks ago

4) ≥ 1: 1024   → 3 weeks ago

CHAPTER 12.

KT DONOR EVALUATION AND MANAGEMENT

I. Deceased donor

1. Donor graft function estimation

1) Age

2) Co-morbidity : DM, HTN (duration)

3) Cause of death

4) Current kidney function : serum Cr. level, urine output.

5) Donor kidney ultrasonography : size, cortical thickness

2. Donor categorization

1) ECD (UNOS criteria)

   (1) Donor age > 60 or

   (2) Donor age 50~59 + two of below

① Terminal serum Cr level > 1.5 mg/dl

② Death by cerebrovascular accident

③ History of HTN

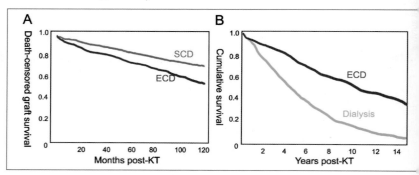

☞ Figure (A) : ECD의 kidney graft를 사용하는 경우 SCD graft에 비하여 long term outcome이 나쁘다(Querard et al., Transpl Int 2016, 29(4): 403-415). 하지만, Figure (B) 에서 보다시피 투석만 하는 경우에 비하여 생존률이 더 높다

(Lloveras et al., Transplantation 2015, 99(5): 991-996).

2) Dual kidney donation candidate (KONOS criteria)

(1) Donor age ≥ 70 + one of below

① Serum Cr level > 3.0 mg/dl and no improvement

② eGFR < 30 mL/min and no improvement

(2) Refused for Standard KT

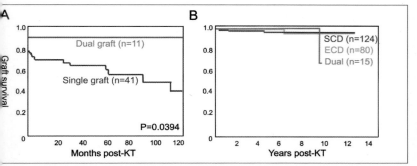

☞ Figure (A) : 75세 이상의 donor에서 kidney graft를 구득하는 경우 dual KT가 더 좋은 성적을 보여줄 수 있다(Gallinat et al., Transplantation 2011, 92(1): 76-81).

Figure (B) : 본원의 Dual KT 성적에서도 유사한 결과를 보여주고 있다.

3) KDRI & KDPI

    (1) 보다 정확하고 객관적인 donor quality assess를 위한 tool로 제시됨.

    (2) Age, Ht, Wt, Race, HTN, DM, Cause of death, serum Cr level, HCV status, DCD KDRI (Continuous score) ⇨ KDPI (%)

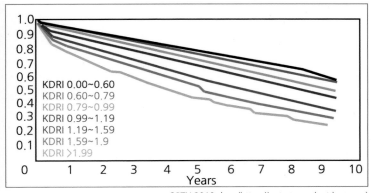

OPTN 2019 data (https://optn.transplant.hrsa.gov)

II. Living donor

1. Laboratory examination

1) Routine Lab

   (1) ABO/Rh typing & Ab screen (T&S)

   (2) HLA-A, B, DR, DQ DNA Typing

   (3) HLA Crossmatch, donor

   (4) CBC with diff, Chemistry, electrolyte, PT/aPTT, HbA1C

   (5) UA c micro., Urine culture, 24hrs urine chemistry, Stool Exam
       Protein/Creatinine Ratio, Albumin/Creatinine Ratio

   (6) Chest PA, EKG, Abdomen Supine/Erect (if needed)

   (7) If DM, Insulin, C-peptide (serum)

2) Evaluation for Infectious Disease

   (1) Hepatitis: HBsAg, anti-HBs, anti-HBc (IgG), anti-HCV

   (2) Others: RPR, Quantitative, anti-HIV, Quantiferon-TB

   (3) Viral serologic status: CMV (IgG), EBV-VCA (IgG), EBNA, EBV
       -EA, VZV Antibody (IgG), Toxoplasma Antibody (IgG)
       HSV (Herpes simplex virus 1,2) Antibody IgG

1. Donation site decision

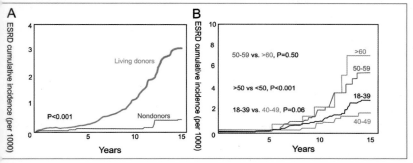

☞ Donor nephrectomy 후에는 일반 건강한 non-donor에 비하여 ESRD의 risk 가 높아짐(Muzaale et al., JAMA. 2014;311(6):579-586).

1) Kidney donation 후 end stage renal disease (ESRD)로 진행할 위험성은 건강한 non-donor에 비하여 높아지며, 그 위험성은 donor의 연령이 많을수록 높아진다.

2) 그렇기 때문에 적절한 donor의 선정은 매우 중요하며, donor의 나이, 기저 질환 그리고 잔존 kidney 의 volume등을 고려하여 donor의 적합성 및 기증할 신장의 좌우를 결정하게 된다.

2. CT angiography

1) Check for specific abnormality : Renal stone, vasculitis or other renal findings

2) Check vasculature and volume of kidney
   : decide Rt. or Lt. nephrectomy, decide open or laparo-scopic nephrectomy

3) Donor safety를 위하여 volume이 작은 kidney를 공여하는 것을 우선 고려한다. 하지만 혈관상태등의 문제도 고려하여 어느 쪽 신장을

공여할지 결정한다.

☞ Some donors show impaired renal adaptation and low e-GFR after nephrectomy. Small residual kidney volume of pre-op CT angiography is associated with decreased post-op 1-month e-GFR , and may lead to impaired renal adaptation.

(Kwon et al, transplantation proc 2017, 49, 1999)

3. Kidney DTPA GFR

1) Check for functional GFR

2) Large cyst 등과 같은 문제로 인하여 CT angiography가 cortical volume을 잘 반영하지 못하는 경우 참조한다.

4. Consultation

1) 정신과 : 『장기 등 기증자 및 장기 등 이식 대기자의 신체검사 항목』 중 살아있는 사람으로서 장기 등 기증 시 정신건강의학과 진료항목 신설. 2012.8.22 일부터 시행

2) 부인과 : 여성인 경우 해당(필요 시)

3) 사회사업팀 : 상담평가를 위한 협진

5. 기증자 지문등록

장기 등 이식에 관한 법률 제 19조에 따라 상담 평가 및 본인 여부 확인을 위해 시행하며 장기이식센터, 사회사업팀, 수술장에서 확인

6. 장기이식관리센터(KONOS)로부터 수술 전 승인을 받는다.

CHAPTER 13.

KIDNEY TRANSPLANTATION PROCEDURE

I. Donor nephrectomy

1. Living donor (Hand Assisted Laparoscopic or Pure laparoscopic surgery)

- Lt. kidney nephrectomy : HALS의 경우 umbilicus의 위쪽으로 midline을 7~8 cm incision 넣어 operator의 좌측 손이 들어간다. 손으로 kidney의 위치를 촉지한 후 umbilicus와 Lt. ASIS를 있는 가상의 선을 기준으로 대칭되게 LLQ에 Scope용 12 mm port를, LUQ에 12 mm acting port를 뚫는다. Pure laparoscopic surgery 의 경우 HALS midline 대신 가장 upper site에 12mm trocar를 insertion하여 operator의 Lt. hand instrument를 넣는다. Graft는 Pfannenstiel incision 을 통해 꺼낸다.

- Rt. kidney nephrectomy : HALS의 경우 Rt. paramedian으로 총 7~8 cm incision을 넣으며 kidney 위치를 고려하여 RUQ에 scope용 12 mm port를, Rt. subcostal area에 12 mm acting port를 뚫는다. 필요 시 liver traction용으로 assist가 사용할 5 mm trocar를 더 위쪽 RUQ-subcostal site에 insertion 한다. Pure laparoscopic surgery 시 HALS midline 대신 가장 lower site에 12 mm trocar를 삽입한다.

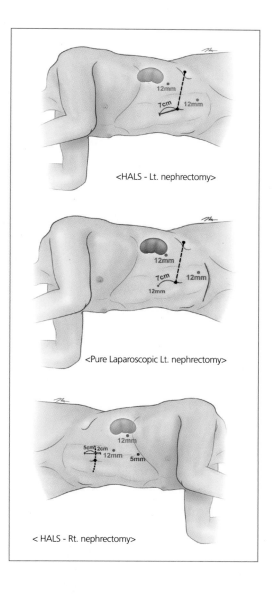

<HALS - Lt. nephrectomy>

<Pure Laparoscopic Lt. nephrectomy>

< HALS - Rt. nephrectomy>

2. Deceased donor

* 수술 전 work up 이 되어 있으면 CT를 확인 후 renal vasculature를 확인해 둔다.

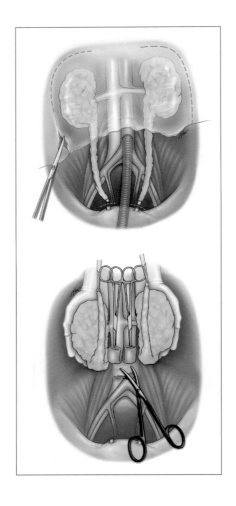

① Deceased donor에서 Perfusion이 끝난 이후 Infrarenal aorta에 cannulation이 되어있는 상태로 catheter 등을 제거하여 field를 정리 한다.

② Iliac fossa 쪽의 retroperitoneum을 조심스럽게 절개, 박리하며 Rt. ureter를 trace하여 bladder 직전까지 확보한 후 ureter를 division 하여 mosquito로 tip을 물어 둔다. Iliac vessel은 후에 extension 용으로 사용해야 할 수 있으므로 조심히 박리한다.

③ Sigmoid colon mobilization 후 Lt. ureter도 마찬가지로 박리하여 division 한다.

④ Kidney를 손으로 받쳐 medial side로 밀면서 kidney 주위의 retroperitoneum을 충분히 넓게 절개를 하고 kidney lateral, posterior, upper side를 박리한다. Upper side는 adrenal gland를 가르는 level까지 올라가면 된다.

⑤ Kidney 하방의 Aorta 및 IVC를 division 후 mosquito로 잡아 놓아 ureter와 함께 상방으로 올리며 다치지 않도록 한다.

⑥ Assistant가 양손으로 kidney, ureter, IVC, Aorta를 모두 끌어안듯이 잡아서 올리면 vertebra의 앞면을 따라 Metzenbaum scissors로 박리를 한다.

⑦ Renal vein보다 상방의 IVC를 가능하다면 여유 있게 division 하고 Aorta는 SMA level에서 division 하면 안전하다.

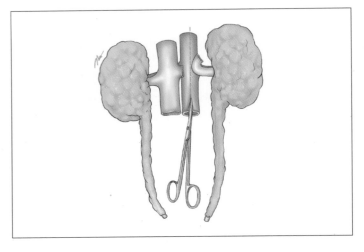

⑧ 양쪽 Kidney가 박리되어 나오면 먼저 IVC 앞면을 조심스럽게 박리하여 Lt. renal vein을 찾은 후 IVC 면에 붙여서 vein을 division 한다. Lt. renal vein이 충분히 좌측으로 젖혀진 것을 확인한 후 Aorta로 잘라야 renal vein이 손상 받지 않을 수 있다.

⑨ Renal artery의 variation 을 주의하며 Aorta 앞쪽 Wall을 정가운데서 Scissors로 자른다. Aorta 내부에서 양측 renal artery로 가는 hole을 확인한 후 Aorta의 후면은 양측 vertebral artery의 사이를 가르면서 정가운데로 절개를 하여 각각의 kidney를 분리한다.

II. Backtable Procedure

1. Perfusion with preservation solution in LDKT

① Donor anatomy를 미리 확인하고 artery, vein 개수와 주행을 확인한다.

② Artery가 직경이 크게 두 개 이상 나올 경우 미리 HTK solution을 2 pack, cannula도 2개 준비하여 필요 시 두 개의 artery에 동시에

perfusion 할 수 있도록 한다. Artery size가 작을 경우 cannula 끝의 tip
이 안 들어갈 수 있으므로 angio cath를 준비한다.

③ Kidney가 나왔을 때 renal vein에 stapler line이 물려 있는 경우
vein 양측 끝을 assistant가 forcep으로 잡도록 하여 stapler가 물려있
는 부분은 scissors로 자르고, renal artery에 cannula tip을 넣은 후
perfusion을 시작한다.

④ Small polar artery가 있을 경우 따로 준비한 HTK solution을 IMA
needle or angiocath로 perfusion 시켜준다.

2. Benchwork

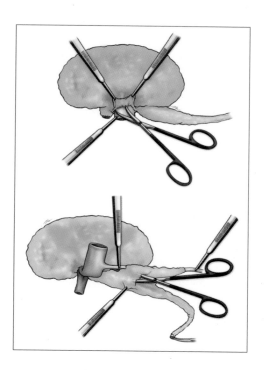

① Rt. kidney일 경우 renal vein이 짧을 수 있으므로 길이 확인 및 recipient의 external iliac vein까지 연결이 가능할지 고려하여 필요 시 저장되어 있는 cryopreserved iliac vein을 준비한다(없을 경우 gonadal vein extension 고려, DDKT 시 IVC 이용을 고려).

② Vein 주위의 fat 및 tissue를 dissection 하면서 anastomosis site를 확보한다. Renal vein으로 drain 되는 small vein (lumbar, adrenal, gonadal 등)에 clipping이 되어있을 경우 tie or suture 해주고 clip은 제거한다. hilum 깊게까지 dissection 할 필요는 없다. Artery도 마찬가지로 dissection 한다.

③ Gonadal vein의 proximal과 distal을 assistant에게 잡고 들어올리게 하고 gonadal vein과 ureter 사이의 plane을 찾아 박리한다. 이때 gonadal vein과 ureter 사이는 tie 하면서 박리한 후 gonadal vein과 불필요한 tissue는 제거한다(필요 시 gonadal vein은 잘 박리하여 extension 용으로 plasty 한다).

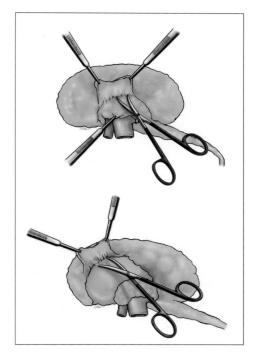

④ Hilum 주위의 fat과 hilum에서 먼 쪽의 fat의 양상이 다름을 확인한
후 그 사이를 경계로 dissection 해서 peripheral 쪽을 removal 해야
한다. 남는 쪽의 fat은 tie한다.

* 가끔씩 fat 안에 polar artery가 숨어있는 경우가 있으니(특히 upper
polar) 수술 전 확인 한 donor CT를 참고하여 artery를 자르지 않도록
조심해야 한다.

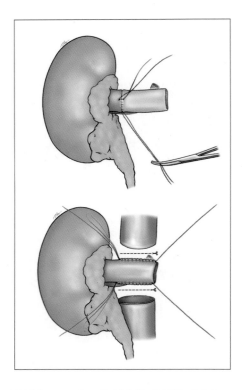

⑤ LDKT의 경우 Rt. Kidney를 사용할 때 병원 내에 Cryopreserved iliac
vein이 보관되어 있을 경우 이용하여 vein extension을 할 수 있다.
valve, size 등을 확인하여 방향에 맞게 anastomosis 하는데 recipient
에 kidney를 넣었을 때 growth factor가 anterior 쪽으로 나오도록
anastomosis를 해주어야 한다(re-perfusion 후 bleeding 시 control
용이).

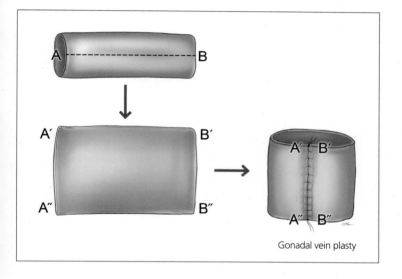

Gonadal vein plasty

⑥ 사용할 수 있는 Cryopreserved iliac vein이 없는 경우, donor
의 gonadal vein이 크기가 적당하면 venoplasty 하여 renal vein
extension 용으로 쓸 수 있다.

⑦ DDKT의 경우 Rt. Kidney를 사용할 때, renal vein의 길이가 짧을 경
우 다양한 방법으로 renal vein을 extension 할 수 있다. 하나의 예
시로 IVC의 상, 하방을 division 후 상기 부위를 suture ligation 하여
hole을 하나로 만들어 줄 수 있다. IVC를 자를 때 쫙 펴서 renal vein
에 너무 가깝게 자르면 자르고 난 후 vein 모양이 오목하게 들어가 좁
아질 위험이 있으므로 주의한다.

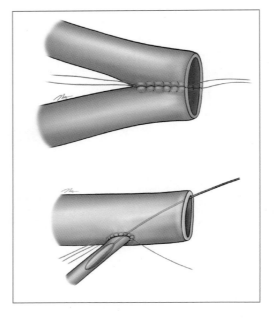

⑧ Multiple artery의 경우, artery의 크기에 따라 side to side anastomosis 또는 end to side anastomosis를 미리 해서 recipient artery와의 anastomosis를 용이하게 할 수 있다.

III. Recipient preparation

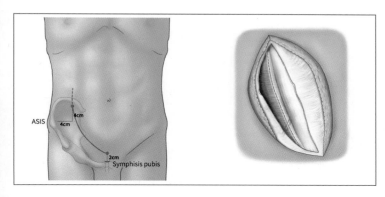

① Symphysis pubis에서 약 1 finger (2 cm) 상방 되는 지점과 및 ASIS에
서 2 finger (4 cm) superior & medial side 되는 지점을 표시한 후 두
지점을 포물선으로 연결하는 hockey stick incision을 넣는다. 위측으
로 가면서는 midline과 평행하게(Rectus muscle의 lateral border 쪽)
으로 배꼽보다 약간 위쪽까지 incision을 넣는다.

② Skin, subcutaneous layer, external fascia까지 dissection을 한 후 보
이는 rectus muscle과 external oblique muscle 사이의 경계로 접근
을 하면 peritoneum을 medial side에서 만날 수 있다.

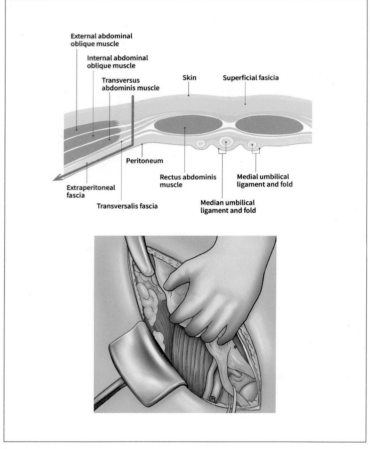

③ Peritoneum이 손상되지 않도록 손으로 밀면서 Psoas muscle을 landmark 삼아 dissection을 진행하면 iliac artery 와 vein까지 도달할 수 있다. 그 후 Bookwalter retractor를 적용한다.

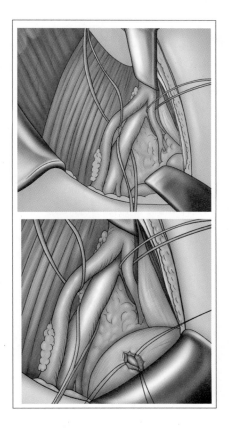

④ Internal and external iliac artery를 촉지하여 상태를 확인한 후 어
  느 쪽을 사용할 건지 정한 후에 상기 artery와 external iliac vein 주
  위를 dissection 하여 anastomosis 하기에 용이하게 만든다. 경우에 따
  라 internal iliac vein을 미리 묶고 잘라주어야 external iliac vein이
  anastomosis한 후 tension 이 걸리지 않을 수 있다.

⑤ Vessel dissection이 끝나고 아래쪽 retractor로 Rectus muscle을

medial side로 충분히 retraction 한 후 bladder muscosa를 찾아 bladder muscle를 dissection 한다. Methylene blue와 Antibiotics를 mix한 용액을 수술 전 미리 bladder에 채워 넣어 놓아야 mucosa가 파란빛으로 보이는 것을 확인할 수 있다.

⑥ 추후 anastomosis를 위한 시야를 확보하기 위해 bladder muscle은 suture하여 mosquito로 물어서 세 방향으로 당겨줄 수 있게 한다.

IV. Transplantation

※ Recipeint의 iliac artery의 상태(주로 calcification 여부) 및 graft의 artery 개수와 모양에 따라 다양한 형태의 anastomosis를 시행할 수 있다.

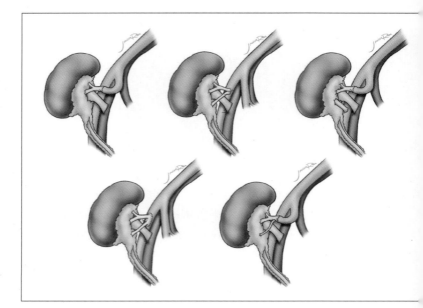

※ Ureter는 bladder muscosa에 먼저 anastomosis를 한 후 bladder muscle
을 다시 덮어주어 leakage를 예방하는 uretero-neocystostomy방법으로
연결할 수 있다.

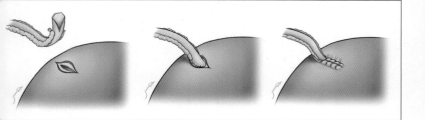

CHAPTER 14.

POST KT MANAGEMENT

I. Post-operative management of Kidney transplantation

1. Immediate Postoperative care

1) Doppler USG

: At POD# 1,3,7 – check for renal vasculature or hydronephrosis

2) DTPA (Renal scan)

: At POD#5-7 – check for ureteral stricture or leakage

3) POD#7 examinations

Examinations	Comment
CBC with Differential	
Chemistry profile	
Electrolyte	

Lipid profile	
Routine UA	
Microscopy, urine	
CMV antigenemia	
Parvovirus B19 Quan. PCR	
Polyomavirus type BK DNA, detection, urine	
Urine (voided)	Check decoy cell
HHV-6 detection (PCR)	
HLA Ab Single Identification, PRA class I	
HLA Ab Single Identification, PRA class II	

4) In case of post-op rejection within 2 weeks

: check HLA Ab Single Identification, PRA class I & II

5) In case of anemia (Hb<7 g/dL)

: check Parvovirus B19

2. Management of Re-admitted recipient (due to elevated serum creatinine)

1) Differential diagnosis

(1) R/O UTI

(2) R/O Dehydration with co-morbid disease

(3) R/O Acute rejection

(4) R/O Viral infection (involve graft)

2) Examinations

(1) CBC with Diff., BUN/ Cr, electrolyte, CRP

(2) UA with micro. Urine Gram stain and culture

(3) BST

(4) Kidney Doppler US

(5) CMV antigenemia

(6) Urine: Decoy cell

(7) Parvovirus B19 Quantitation. PCR (blood)

(8) Polyomavirus type BK (Urine)

(9) HHV-6 detection PCR

(10) Kidney Biopsy

    ① R/O Rejection

    ② R/O Viral infection: CMV, BK virus

II. Out-Patient follow-up

1. Follow up frequency

- before post-operative 1 month : every 1-2 weeks
- after 1 month : every 1 month f/u

2. Routine Lab at OPD

1) CBC with differential

2) Chemistry profile, Electrolyte Profile, Lipid Profile

3) Routine Urinalysis, Microscopy, Urine

4) Tacrolimus or Cyclosporin, Mycophenolic Acid

5) CMV antigenemia

6) Urine (void) - Decoy cell

7) Urine Protein/Creatinine ratio

   Urine Albumin/Creatinine ratio

8) Protein, 24hr Urine, CCr (Creatinine Clearance)

   (check at 12 weeks, 20 weeks, 6 moths, 1 year, then yearly)

3. HLA Ab Single Identification, class I &II

1) Check at pre-op work-up, post op 1 week, 4 week, 1 year, and annually

4. Virus panels : check at postop 1, 5, 9, 16, 24 weeks

1) HHV-6 Detection PCR

2) Parvovirus B19 DNA, detection

   ① Positive → Parvovirus B19 DNA, Quantitation

3) Urine Polyomavirus type BK DNA, detection [PCR]

   ① Positive → urine Polyomavirus type BK DNA quantitation

   Whole blood Polyomavirus type BK DNA quantitation, WB

   * Chapter 3 INFECTION IN TRANSPLANT RECIPIENTS 참고

5. Post-op 1 year exams

1) Hepatitis Profile/anti-HCV Antibody

2) 24hr Urine protein & CCr (Creatinine Clearance)

3) EGD/ Colonoscopy

4) Bone Whole body Scan

5) Bone Densitometry

6) Transplanted Renal Doppler US

7) HLA Ab Single Identification, class I &II

8) Chest-PA&Lat, EKG

9) Breast US, Mammography (female only)

10) OBGY, cancer screening (female only)

6. Other medications

Name	Usage	Comment
Sulfamethoxxazole/Trimethoprim	1T qd	Discontinue at post-op 6 months
Esomeprazole	1T qd	
Diomagnite	1 Pack HS	
Chlorhexidin gargle	frequently	

※ Aspirin (ASPC): discontinue at post-op 1 year, if taking

7. Target levels for DM and HTN control

1) Hb A1C   <7%

2) Fasting glucose   <130 mg/dL

3) Blood pressure   <130/80 mmHg

4) LDL-cholesterol   <100 mg/dL

CHAPTER 15.

KIDNEY TRANSPLANTATION PROTOCOL

I. Immunosuppression protocol

1. rATG induction (rabbit Anti-thymocyte Globulin)

1) General Concept

(1) 2nd or ECD-DDKT, expected an immediate delayed graft function

(2) Use in High or intermediate Immunologic risk cases.

(3) With Methylprednisolone 500 mg IV (intra-op.)

(4) 1.5 mg/kg over 12hrs (POD # 0 ~ 2 for 3 days) through central line

(5) CMV prophylaxis : ganciclovir 5 mg/kg iv q 24hr for 2 weeks

(6) Fungal prophylaxis : itraconazole 100 mg bid for 2 weeks

2) Maintenance immunosuppression

(1) Tacrolimus & MMF : administered from POD#1 afternoon

(2) Steroids are tapered according to schedule

2. Basiliximab induction (IL-2 receptor blocker)

1) General Concept

   (1) Low immunologic risk cases or SCD-DDKT

   (2) With Methylprednisolone 500 mg IV (intra-op.)

   (3) Use intra-op and POD#4

2) Maintenance Immunosuppressant

   (1) Tacrolimus & MMF : administered from POD#0 afternoon

   (2) Steroids are tapered according to schedule

3. Maintenance

1) Target Trough Level of Tacrolimus

   (1) OP ~ 2 weeks : around 10 ng/mL

   (2) 2 weeks ~ 1 month : 8-10 ng/mL

   (3) After 1 month : 5-8 ng/mL

2) Target Trough Level of Cyclosporin

   (1) Up to 1 month : 150-200 ng/mL

   (2) 1 month ~ 3 months : 100-150 ng/mL

   (3) After 3 months : 100 ng/mL

3) Prednisolone (Methylprednisolone)

   (1) POD# 8 Start up to 2 weeks 16 mg bid

   (2) after 2 weeks : Maintain 8 mg bid until 4 weeks

   (3) Keep 4 mg bid for 5 to 12 weeks then give 4 mg qd.

4) MMF

   (1) Start with tacrolimus

   (2) Side effect : Diffuse abdominal pain or diarrhea, leukopenia

   (3) If patient suffer severe GI trouble, consider changing to Mycophenolic acid

II. Peripoperative fluid management

1. Post-transplantation fluid Replacement

  1) Post Op- day & POD#1

    (1) Main fluid (Half saline 1 L) : 80 cc/hr

    (2) SOW start

    (3) Urine replacement

Hourly urine	Replace
<50 mL	Notify Dr.
50-100	150%
100-200	120%
200-300	100%
300-500	80%
>500	60%

  2) POD#2

    (1) Main fluid (Half saline 1 L) : 80 cc/hr

    (2) SBD start

    (3) Urine replacement

Hourly urine	Replace
<50 mL	Notify Dr.
50-100	120%

100-200	100%
200-300	80%
>300	60%

3) POD# 3

   (1) Replace Hold, Keep vein with Half saline 2 L (80 cc/hr)

4) POD# 4

   (1) Keep vein with Half saline 2 L (80 cc/hr)

III. Perioperative antimicrobial management

1. Antibiotics

1) Day 0 ~ 2 : Cefotaxime IV 2.0 g q8hrs

   In case of r-ATG induction, use cefotaxime until POD # 4

2. INH prophylaxis if required

1) INH 300 mg, B6 50 mg / day for 9 months (if active tuberculosis history (+))

3. CMV prophylaxis

1) Use when induction with r-ATG induction

2) IV Ganciclovir for 2 weeks

3) If CMV D+/R-: IV Ganciclovir for 2 weeks, PO valganciclovir 900 mg qd for 200days

4. HBs Ag (+) recipient

1) Consultation to hepatologist and start anti-viral agent after transplantation.

IV. Other Drugs

1. Anti-hypertensive agents (Prn. order after operation)

1) If BP > 160/90, Start Nifedipine 30 mg qd

2) If BP continued higher, use Nifedipine 60 mg bid, Carvedirol 25 mg bid or 50 mg bid

3) If intractable, consult to Cardiologist

2. Alprostadil injection

1) Keep patent arterial flow after anastomosis

2) 투여대상: 신장이식 환자(① ~ ③ 중 한개 만족시)

　　① Cadaveric donor kidney (ECD Kidney 등)

　　② Microvessel anastomosis가 필요한 신이식 수술 환자

　　③ Acute rejection 가능성이 높은 환자(아래 4개 중 한개 만족시)

　　　- HLA mismatching환자

　　　- PRA (Panel Reactive Anti-body) > 30%인 환자

　　　- ABO mismatching

　　　- Retransplantation of Kidney

3) 재투여 기준: 동맥재건술을 재시행해야 하는 경우

4) 투여중단 기준: Adverse effect 또는 과민반응이 나타난 경우 (ex. 혈압 하강시)

V. Rejection protocol

1. Steroid pulse therapy

1) Bolus Methylprednisolone 500 mg IV : for 3 days

2) Followed by a short steroid recycle → reduce daily half dose

　　(1) 500-500-500-250-125-75-60 mg

(2) From 8th day MPD 16 mg bid for 3 days, 8 mg bid for 3 days, 4 mg bid for 3 days, maintain 4 mg qd until OPD

3) Use SMX-TMP 1T QD daily, total 6 weeks.

2. rATG, Intra Venous Immune Globulin (IVIG) Therapy

- Chapter 02. IMMUNOSUPPRESSION PROTOCOL 참고(26, 41pg).

VI. Desensitization protocol according to immunologic risk group

1. Immunologic risk stratification

1) High risk : meet one of the requirements below $\Rightarrow$ admission 2 weeks ago

   (1) Positive HLA crossmatching (CDC;complement-dependent cytotoxicity)

   (2) Positive HLA flow cytometry crossmatch (FCXM)

   (3) Positive DSA and DSA MFI $\geq$ 2500

2) Intermediate risk :

   Positive DSA and DSA MFI < 2500

3) Low risk : negative DSA, PRA (Luminex) is irrelevant.

2. SMC protocol for desensitization

1) High risk : Plasmapheresis (PP)/IVIG #5 + Rituximab + rATG

   (1) Rituximab (375 mg/m^2) administered one month before transplantation

   (2) Plasmapheresis every other day $\rightarrow$ IVIG 200 mg/kg the day after PP

(3) Post-PP lab (fibrinogen, PT/aPTT, albumin, protein).

(4) When performing plasmapheresis, DFPP (double filtration PP) or TPE (therapeutic plasma exchange) should be performed differently depending on the patient's condition.

(5) The last two PP must be replaced with FFP before transplantation.

(6) Primary endpoint : CDC-CXM (-)

(7) if FCXM (+) → FCXM test at 1 day before transplantation

　　→ perform operation according to clinician's decision

　　　if DSA MFI≥2500 → HLA Ab single, class I or II at 1 day before transplantation → perform operation according to clinician's decision

2) Intermediate risk: Rituximab (375 mg/m^2) (POD#-2)+ rATG

3) Low risk: No desensitization is needed (basiliximab induction).

VII. ABO incompatible Kidney Transplantation

1. Rituximab

1) One month before surgery

2) Admission schedule according to the ABO isoagglutinin titer

　(1) ≤1: 32　　　　　→ 7 days ago

　(2) 1: 64 ~ 1: 128　→ 10 days ago

　(3) ≥1: 256　　　　→ 2 weeks ago

　(4) ≥1: 1024　　　　→ 3 weeks ago

3) Dose: Initial titer

　(1) ≥1: 256　　　　→ 375 mg/m^2

　(2) ≤1: 128　　　　→ 200 mg

4) Admission (usually friday), before administration titer/crossmatch/ PRA check!!

2. Immunosuppression

1) Induction: r-ATG (POD #0,1,2)

2) Tacrolimus & MMF : POD# -7 start, Tacrolimus target level is 8 before operation

    Tacrolimus target level is 10 after operation

3. Plasmapheresis

1) Ab titer → use Monospecific AHG IgG phase

2) Target pre-OP Ab titer → 1: 32

3) If the initial Ab titer is 1: 256 or more

    (1) Preoperative IVIG use

      ① Dose: 200 mg/kg

      ② Schecdule: consider every day or every other day

      ③ Timing: Give 1-2 hours after Plasmapheresis, give the next day in some cases. It is recommended to take PP for one day after IVIG administration, since giving IVIG and then PP can be clearing. The important thing is to use IVIG after PP

    (2) Start with EOD PP

    (3) If 1: 32 is not reached, daily PP is performed. If 3 consecutive titer values are maintained, consider operation.

4) If Ab titer is less than 1: 256, no IVIG, EOD PP only

4. Postoperative management

1) POD#1~#14: check titier daily → Consideration of PP in case of 3 or more rises compared to titer just before transplantation (compared to titer of POD #-1)

2) POD#15~#30: weekly check

3) Protocol biopsy at POD#12

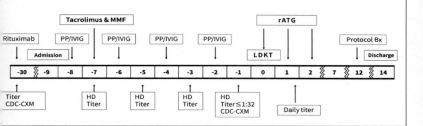

LDKT Preoperative (- 2 day) order

1. Check V/S q 8hrs
2. WA
3. CRF diet
4. Check I/O, Body Weight
5. 0.1% chlorhexidine solution gargle q 6h
6. Get Op. permission
   * medications *
7. Esomeprazole 1T PO BID
8. Diogel 1 pack PO HS
9. Continue maintenance antihypertensive drug, diuretics, antibiotics
10. Check transplantation work up list.
   1) HLA cross matching Check results
   2) Anti HIV, EBV, CMV, HSV antibody test,
      HBs Ag, HBs Ab, HBe Ag, HBe Ab, HBc Ab,HCV Ab
      If HBsAg (+) → check HBV DNA Quantitation,
      check HBeAg/HBeAb. HBcAb
      If Anti-HCV (+) → check HCV RNA detection (PCR)
   3) History Check
      Check HD or CAPD, check dialysis hospital
      CRF treatment period - Underlying renal disease
      Check Bladder capacity, Reflux level
      Check for recent infection sign- Check Dental, ENT consult
      Check Donor relationship
11. Check Donor CT angiography results (Polar artery): Which Kidney to use
12. Laboratory test
   1) CBC with platelet count
   2) coagulation profile
   3) liver profile
   4) electrolyte, BUN, Cr
   5) Sputum, urine, and throat swab for bacterial, and fungal culture
   6) Nasal MRSA, VRE rectal screening

LDKT Preoperative (- 1 day) order

1. Check V/S q 8hrs
2. WA
3. CRF diet → from 5PM NPO
4. Check I/O, body Weight at 6AM
5. 0.1% chlorhexidine solution gargle q 6hr
6. Send the patient to Hemodialysis Unit
   (check electrolyte, BUN, Cr., after dialysis)
7. Esomeprazole 1T PO BID
8. Diogel 1 pack PO HS
9. Continue maintenance antihypertensive drug, diuretics, antibiotics
10. 5 DW half saline 1 L
11. Blood Type and Crossmatch
12. Duplex sonography, carotid
    L/E artery (bilateral) duplex
    If have a problem -- consult to Dept. of Anesthesiology
13. Prepare package
    Ward preparation: Cefotaxime 2 g. x 3 (with AST)
    Basiliximab 1 vial prep.
    Anti-embolic DVT cuff: prep

Preoperative adult Kidney Transplantation orders (Operative Day)

1. Check V/S q 8 hrs
2. BR
3. NPO except for medication
4. Check I/O q 4 h, body weight at 6AM
5. Elastic antiembolic stocking at OR
6. 0.1% Chlorohexidine solution gargling q 6h
7. Half saline1000 mL IV
8. Skin test for cefotaxime
9. Premedication (by anesthesiologist)
10. Famotidine 1V IVS on 6AM
11. Diabetics : BST q 2h until OR with RI continuous scale as follows

Blood glucose	RI continuous injection (unit/hr)
150 - 200	0
201 - 250	1
251 - 300	2
301 - 350	3
> 350	4, call Dr.

12. Send the patient to OR on call with package
    : Prepare Disposable anti-embolic cuff for DVT prevention.
13. In case of DDKT, prepare S-B, formalin tube (for zero time biopsy)

DDKT Preoperative order

1. Check V/S q 8h
2. WA
3. NPO
4. Check I/O, Body Weight
5. 0.1% chlorhexidine solution gargle q 6h
6. Get Op. permission

   * medications *

7. Famotidine 1V ivs
8. Continue maintenance antihypertensive drug, diuretics, antibiotics
9. Check transplantation work up list.

   1) HLA cross matching Check results
   2) Anti HIV, EBV, CMV, HSV antibody test,

      HBs Ag, HBs Ab, HBe Ag, HBe Ab, HBc Ab,HCV Ab

      If HBsAg (+) → check HBV DNA Quantitation,

      check HBeAg/HBeAb. HBcAb

      If Anti-HCV (+) → check HCV RNA detection (PCR)
   3) History Check

      Check HD or CAPD, check dialysis hospital

      CRF treatment period - Underlying renal disease

      Check Bladder capacity, Reflux level

      Check for recent infection sign-

      Check Dental, ENT consult

      Check Donor relationship

10. Laboratory *

    1) CBC with platelet count
    2) coagulation profile
    3) liver profile
    4) electrolyte, BUN, Cr
    5) Sputum, urine, and throat swab for bacterial, and fungal culture
    6) Nasal MRSA, VRE rectal screening
    7) PRA Ab single Identification (Class I, II)
    8) Chest PA
    9) PNS series
    10) Spirometry and F/V curve
    11) Advanced echo
    12) Duplex scan, Carotid
    13) Duplex scan, L/E Artery (bilateral)
    14) Abdomen and pelvis CT (non-contrast)

Intraoperative orders for adult Kidney Transplantation recipient

1. Foley catheter, 18F male, 20F female
2. Bladder irrigation fluid culture
3. Gentamicin solution: instill to the bladder approximately 150-300 mL by gravity and clamp Foley with two Kelly clamps
   (Gentamicin solution: GM 80 mg in 1,000 mL saline with 10 drop of indigocarmin)
4. Ensure that preoperative antibiotic administered.
   Cefotaxime 2 g IV Side
5. Antiembolic stockings & Vascular Refilling Detector
6. Diabetes: blood glucose monItoring to keep blood glucose 150±25
7. Patient should be well hydrated before revascularization
   CVP should be 12-16 or patient should receive at least 2500 mL during anesthesia
8. Induction of Immunosuppression with Basiliximab 1a IV or rATG 1.5 mg/kg IV
9. When arterial anastomosis begins:
   lasix 40 mg IV
   Mannitol 1 gm per kg IV
   Methylprednisolone 500 mg IVS
   ensure patient is well hydrated
10. After the operation, ensure both femoral pulses are present and strong
    Check the feet also.

POSTOP kidney transplantation protocol

1. Check V/S q 1hr with monitoring
2. BR with Semi-Fowler's position & Rt.hip flexion and leg elevation
3. NPO except medication
4. Check I/O q 4hr (hourly urine check)
5. Check Bwt
6. CVP monitoring q 4hr
7. Keep foley in situ with natural drainage
8. Cough & deep breath q 2hr & incentive spirometer q 1hr while awake
9. Anti-embolic stockings & vascular refilling detector until POD#2
10. Check bilateral lower extremity pulses q 4hr
11. Avoid IM injection on right buttock
12. 0.1% Chlorohexidine solution gargling q 8hr
13. BST q 6hr
   : If Blood Glucose Level (BGL) <100 or >240, △BGL >80 → recheck 2hrs later
   1) **Initiation**
      (1) 160 mg/dl< BGL < 240 mg/dl → starting rate: 1unit/hr
      (2) 240 mg/dl < BGL ⇨ starting rate: 2unit/hr
   2) ** Maintenance**
      (1) BGL < 100 → stop for 2hrs & notify & restart when >180 by rate -1unit/hr
      (2) 100 ≤ BGL < 140 → rate -1units/hr
      (3) 140 ≤ BGL < 160 → maintain rate
      (4) 160 ≤ BGL < 240 → rate +1unit/hr (maintain if BGL is decreasing)
      (5) 240 ≤ BGL < 300 → rate +2unit/hr (maintain if BGL is decreasing)
      (6) 300 ≤ BGL → rate +2unit/hr & notify
14. Half normal saline 1L iv c 40 mL/hr, 5DHN 1 L 40cc/hr
15. Post transplantation solution (Half saline 1 L) replace
    H/U < 50 mL → call Dr.
    50-100 mL → 150%

        100-200 mL → 120%

        200-300 mL → 100%

        300-500 mL → 80%

        >500 mL → 60%

16. CVP replacement with Volulyte.

    If CVP < 4 mmHg → 2 cc/kg/hr → recheck 2hr later

    < 10 mmHg → 1 cc/kg/hr

    10-12 mmHg → stop

17. Cefotaxime 2 g iv q 8hr

18. Alprostadil 1.47 mcg/kg (in NS 50 mL) mivs 4 cc/hr q 12hr

    if microsurgery (or renal artery) or DDKT (total 14 times)

19. Famotidine 1A + NS 50 mL iv q 12hr, Ambroxol 1A, Diogel 1p P HS

20. PRN) Hydromorphone 1 mg iv

21. CBC, e, chemistry, ion Ca, PT/aPTT, S-osm, ABGA, UA c micro, urine (e, osm), Chest AP, ABGA

22. CBC, e, BUN/Cr, S-osm/U-osm q 8hr

23. Prn) Labetalol 10 mg iv / 20% Albumin 100 mL iv (alb<3.0) / Demerol 1A + N/S 50 mL mixed iv

24. If rATG was used, acetaminophen 325 mg po q4hr, chlorpheniramine 1A iv.

KT POD #1

1. Check V/S q 1hr with monitoring
2. BR with Semi-Fowler's position & Rt.hip flexion and leg elevation
3. SOW
4. Check I/O q 8hr (hourly urine check)
5. Check Bwt
6. CVP monitoring q 8hr & replacement with volulyte

    If CVP < 4 mmHg → 2 cc/kg/hr → recheck 2hr later

    < 10 mmHg → 1 cc/kg/hr

    10-12 mmHg → stop

7. Keep foley with natural drainage
8. Cough & deep breath q 2hr & incentive spirometer
9. Anti-embolic stockings until POD#2
10. Check bilateral lower extremity pulses q 4hr
11. Avoid IM injection on right buttock
12. 0.1% Chlorohexidine solution gargling q 8hr
13. 24hr urine collection for Ccr (from 6AM to 6AM) (check of POD # 1, 3, and 5)
14. BST check q 6hr

    :If BGL <100 or >240, △BGL >80 → recheck 2hrs later

    1) ** Initiation **

       (1) 160 mg/dl< BGL < 240 mg/dl → starting rate: 1unit/hr
       (2) 240 mg/dl < BGL → starting rate: 2unit/hr

    2) ** Maintenance **

       (1) BGL< 100 → stop for 2hrs & notify & restart when >180 by rate -1unit/hr
       (2) 100 ≤ BGL < 140 → rate -1units/hr
       (3) 140 ≤ BGL < 160 → maintain rate
       (4) 160 ≤ BGL < 240 → rate +1unit/hr (maintain if BGL is decreasing)
       (5) 240 ≤ BGL < 300 → rate +2unit/hr (maintain if BGL is decreasing)
       (6) 300 ≤ BGL → rate +2unit/hr & notify

15. Half saline 1 L iv c 40 mL/hr, 5DHN 1 L 40 cc/hr

16. Post transplantation solution (Half saline 1 L) replace

    H/U   <50 mL → call Dr.

    50-100 mL   → 120%

    100-200 mL   → 100%

    200-300 mL   → 80%

    >300 mL   → 60%

17. Cefotaxime 2 g iv q 8hr

18. Alprostadil 1.47 mcg/kg (in NS 50 mL, 4 cc/hr) bid if microsurgery or DDKT

19. Famotidine 1A + NS 50 mL iv q 12hr, ambroxol 1A q8hr, Diogel 1p p.o HS

20. Tacrolimus (/) mg po bid or Cyclosporin (/) mg po bid

21. MMF (/) mg p.o bid after confirm

22. Methylprednisolone 500 mg iv q 24hr

23. prn) Morphine 3 mg iv / labetalol 10 mg ivs / Demerol 1A + N/S 100 mL mixed iv

24. CBC, e, chemistry, ion Ca, PT/aPTT, S-osm, Ccr, UA c micro, urine (e, osm), Chest AP at 5AM

25. e, BUN/Cr, S-osm/U-osm at 5PM

26. prn) 5% Albumin 250 mL iv (alb<3.0)

27. Doppler sonography is performed on the POD # 1 day (re-check if there is any special Finding)

28. The DTPA confirms the schedule in advance on the POD # 5-7.

KT POD #2

1. Check V/S q 1hr
2. BR with Semi-Fowler's position & Rt.hip flexion and leg elevation
3. SBD
4. Check I/O q 8hr (hourly urine check)
5. Check Bwt
6. CVP monitoring q 8hr & replacement with volulyte

    If CVP < 4 mmHg → 2 cc/kg/hr → recheck 2hr later

        < 10 mmHg → 1 cc/kg/hr

        10-12 mmHg → stop

7. Keep foley in situ with natural drainage
8. Cough & deep breath q 2hr & incentive spirometer
9. Anti-embolic stockings until ambulation
10. Check bilateral lower extremity pulses q 4hr
11. Avoid IM injection on right buttock
12. 0.1% Chlorohexidine solution gargling q 8hr
13. BST check q 6hr
 1) BST check q6hr (SBD)
 2) BSL 200~250 → RI 4U SC
 3) BSL 251~300 → RI 8U SC
 4) BSL 301~350 → RI 12U SC
 5) BSL>350 or <80 → notify to Dr
14. Half saline 2 L iv c 80 mL/hr
15. Post transplantation solution (Half saline 1 L) replace

    H/U <50 mL   → call Dr.

    50-100 mL   → 120%

    100-200 mL   → 100%

    200-300 mL   → 80%

    >300 mL   → 60%

16. Cefotaxime 2 g iv q 8hr (Prophylactic antibiotics only give up to POD # 2 days)

17. Alprostadil 1.47 mcg/kg (in NS 50 mL, 4 cc/hr) bid if microsurgery or DDKT

18. Esomeprazole 20 mg qd, ambroxol 1T BID

19. Tacrolimus (/) mg po bid or Cyclosporin (/) mg po bid

20. MMF (/) mg p.o bid after confirm

21. Methylprednisolone 250 mg iv q 24hr

22. Diogel 1p p.o HS

23. prn) Labetalol 10 mg ivs / Morphine 5 mg iv (if pain develop)

24. CBC, e, chemistry, ion Ca, PT/aPTT, S-osm, Ccr, UA c micro, Chest AP, tacrolimus level at 5AM

25. e, BUN/Cr, S-osm/U-osm at 5PM

26. prn) 20% alb 100 mL iv(alb<3.0)

    prn) Demerol 1A + N/S 50 mL mixed iv

KT POD #3

1. Check V/S q 1hr
2. BR with Semi-Fowler's position & Rt.hip flexion and leg elevation
3. SBD or NRD
4. Check I/O q 8hr (hourly urine check)
5. Check Bwt
6. CVP monitoring q 8hr
7. Keep foley in situ with natural drainage
8. Anti-embolic stockings until ambulation
9. Avoid IM injection on right buttock
10. 0.1% Chlorohexidine solution gargling q 8hr
11. 24hr urine collection for Ccr (from 6AM to 6AM)
12. BST check q 6hr
    1) BST check q6 hr (SBD)
    2) BSL 200~250 → RI 4U SC
    3) BSL 251~300 → RI 8U SC
    4) BSL 301~350 → RI 12U SC
    5) BSL>350 or <80 → notify to Dr
13. Half saline 2 L (80 cc/hr)
14. Alprostadil 1.47 mcg/kg (in NS 50 mL, 4 cc/hr) bid if microsurgery or DDKT
15. E-poietin SC : EOD injection when Hb < 10 g/dl (If Bwt < 50 kg, inject 4000IU / if ≥ 50 kg, inject 6000IU) until discharge
16. Esomeprazole 20 mg qd, ambroxol 1T BID
17. Tacrolimus (/) mg po bid or Cyclosporin (/) mg po bid
18. MMF (/) mg p.o bid
19. Methylprednisolone 125 mg iv q 24hr
20. Diogel 1p p.o HS
21. prn) Demerol 1A + N/S 50 mL iv
22. CBC, e, chemistry, ion Ca, PT/aPTT, S-osm, Ccr, UA c micro, urine (e, osm), chest AP (p),TDM Tacrolimus (or cyclosporin) at 5AM
23. e, BUN/Cr, S-osm/U-osm at 5PM
24. prn) Labetalol 10 mg iv
25. prn) Lasix 10 mg iv or lasix 20 mg iv
26. prn) Mida 3 mg iv

KT POD #4

1. Check V/S q 4hr
2. BR with Semi-Fowler's position & Rt.hip flexion and leg elevation
3. SBD or NRD
4. Check I/O q 8hr (hourly urine check)
5. Check Bwt
6. Keep foley in situ with natural drainage
7. Anti-embolic stockings until ambulation
8. Avoid IM injection on right buttock
9. 0.1% Chlorohexidine solution gargling q 8hr
10. BST check q 6hr
    1) BST check q6hr (SBD)
    2) BSL 200~250 → RI 4U SC
    3) BSL 251~300 → RI 8U SC
    4) BSL 301~350 → RI 12U SC
    5) BSL>350 or <80 → notify to Dr
11. Half saline 2 L (80 cc/hr)
12. Alprostadil 1.47 mcg/kg (in NS 50 mL, 4 cc/hr) bid if microsurgery or DDKT
13. E-poietin SC : EOD injection when Hb < 10 g/dl (If Bwt < 50 kg, inject 4000IU/ if ≥ 50 kg, inject 6000IU) until discharge
14. Esomeprazole 20 mg p.o qd
15. Basiliximab 20 mg IVs
16. Tacrolimus (/) mg po bid or Cyclosporin (/) mg po bid
17. MMF (/)mg p.o bid
18. Methylprednisolone 75 mg iv q 24hr
19. Diogel 1p p.o HS
20. prn) Morphine 3 mg iv
21. CBC, e, chemistry, ion Ca, PT/aPTT, S-osm, Ccr, UA c micro, urine(e, osm), Chest AP (p), CyA at 5AM
22. e, BUN/Cr, S-osm/U-osm at 5PM
23. Check DTPA.

KT POD #5~7

1. Check V/S q 4hr
2. BR with Semi-Fowler's position & Rt.hip flexion and leg elevation
3. NRD (drink more than 100c of water during 1 hour)
4. check I/O q 8hrs
5. check hour urine
6. check body weight
7. Remove Foley in situ (Check DTPA result before remove)
   Remove 후 1시간에 한 번씩 소변을 보도록 환자 교육, POD #7 부터는 2시간에 한 번 voiding. bladder capacity가 작았던 경우(< 100 cc)에는 며칠간 foley training 하고 괜찮으면 제거.
8. antiembolic stockings until ambulation
9. avoid IM injection on right buttock
10. 0.1% Chlorohexidine solution gargling q 8h
11. collect 24h urine for Ccr
12. Esomeprazol 20 mg qd, Diogel 1T PO
13. Tacrolimus (/) mg po bid or Cyclosporin (/) mg po bid
14. Methylprednisolone 60 mg iv (POD#5,6,7)
15. MMF (/) mg po Bid
16. SMX-TMP 1T qd for 6 months
17. CBC, e, chemistry, ion Ca, PT/aPTT, S-osm, Ccr, UA c micro, urine (e, osm), Chest AP (p), CyA at 5AM
18. e, BUN/Cr, S-osm/U-osm at 5PM
19. Laboratory test after POD # 5
    CBC, E', Bun/Cr & FK or CyA level : daily

chemistry profile, UA with micro, serum Osm/urine Osm (em) : every other day

20. POD# 7 : Routine check Lab
    1) CBC with diff
    2) Chemistry profile, Electrolyte profile, Lipid Profile
    3) Routine Urinalysis, Microscopy, Urine
    4) FK 506 (Tacrolimus) or Cyclosporin, Mycophenolic Acid
    5) CMV antigenemia
    6) Urine (void) – check Decoy cell
    7) Protein/Creatinine, Ratio, Urine, Albumin/Creatinine, Ratio, Urine
    8) HHV-6 Detection PCR
    9) Parvovirus B19 DNA, detection
       If (+), check Parvovirus B19 DNA, Quantitation
    10) Polyomavirus type BK DNA, detection, urine [PCR]
        If (+), check urine and whole blood Polyomavirus type BK DNA, quantitation
    11) Urine, sputum, blood : Bacterial & fungal culture ⇒ POD #7, #14...
21. Alprostadil 1.47 mcg/kg (in NS 50 mL, 4 cc/hr) bid if microsurgery or DDKT
22. E-poietin SC : EOD injection when Hb < 10 g/dl (If Bwt < 50 kg, inject 4000IU / if ≥ 50 kg, inject 6000IU) until discharge
23. Consult to Infectionist part before discharge and make an appoint at Out patient department

⟨ KT basic Schedule ⟩

POD#1 : doppler USG

POD#3 : doppler USG

POD#4 : If there is no abnormality in the Wound, open it and then cover it with Tegaderm.

POD#5 : DTPA

SMX-TMP start (1T qd for 6mon)

POD#6 : Foley remove (after DTPA)

    --- POD#5 & POD#6 : check hourly urination

    -- after POD#7 : About once every 2 hours Urination

POD#7 : doppler USG , C-line remove - alprostadil D/C,

    - Parvovirus, Polyoma virus, HHV-6 etc.. (See the table on the previous page)

    HLA Ab Single Identification, Class I & II

    nutrition, Pharmaceutical department Consult

POD#12 : Protocol kidney bx

POD#14 : Discharge & Stitch out (consult to infectionist before discharge)

POD#21 : Outpatient appointment with infectionist

* In KT patients, rejection occurred within 2 weeks after surgery :
HLA Ab Single Identification, PRA class I HLA Ab Single Identification, PRA class II

< Prescription at first discharge: Examination at KT 3~4 weeks >

- CBC with diff.
- Chemistry profile, Electrolyte profile, Lipid Profile
- Routine Urinalysis, Microscopy, Urine
- Tacrolimus or Cyclosporin, Mycophenolic Acid
- CMV antigenemia
- Protein/Creatinine, Ratio, Urine, Albumin/Creatinine, Ratio, Urine
- HLA Ab Single Identification, PRA class I & II

* Alprostadil

Indication −

    1) DDKT

    2) When microsurgery is used for artery anastomosis, aspirin is prescribed after surgery.

Volume − 1.47 mcg/kg, twice a day

CHAPTER 16.

PANCREAS TRANSPLANTATION MANAGEMENT

I. Recipient management

1. DM co-morbidity

- 최근 연구 결과들에 따르면 pancreas transplantation 이후 glucose control이 normalization 되는 경우 DM의 합병증들이 호전되는 것을 보고하고 있다. 특히 DM nephropathy, retinopathy, neuropathy가 호전되고, cardiovascular event가 감소하며, 결국 mortality rate가 낮아진다. (Jenssen T et al., Curr Opin Organ Transplant 2017, 22(4): 382-388.)

2. Pancreas transplantation complications

1) Vein thrombosis : 가장 흔히 발생할 수 있는 합병증으로 원래 portal vein의 inflow 3방향(SMV, IMV, splenic vein) 중 SMV와 IMV의 flow

가 차단되고 splenic vein의 flow만 남게 되므로 thrombosis가 잘 발생하게 된다(Chapter 17. Bench procedure 그림 6. 참조). 이를 예방하기 위한 여러가지 방법이 제시되고 있으며, 본원에서는 수술 후 heparinization을 시행하고, (Pancreas transplantation protocol chapter 및 appendix. Heparin nomogram를 참조), operator와 상의하여 시작한다. 경구 섭취가 가능해지는 경우는 oral anticoagulation medication으로 변경한다. Post OP day 2, 7에 CT angiography를 check하여 thrombosis 여부를 확인한다

2) Bleeding : thrombosis를 예방하기 위하여 anticoagulation을 시행하고, SMA 주변 connective tissue에 small vessel branch들이 많기 때문에 post OP bleeding의 risk가 높으며, post OP day1 or 2 에 JP color 및 Hb change를 확인하고 anticoagulation 여부를 결정한다. Heparinization을 시작한 이후에도 JP color 및 Hb의 변화를 주의해서 봐야한다.

3) Exocrine leakage : pancreas graft에는 endocrine function (insulin) 뿐만 아니라, exocrine function (amylase, lipase) 도 가지고 있으며, 이를 어떻게 drain하는가가 중요한 문제이다. 최근에는 enteric drainage를 선호하고 있으며, 본원에서는 duodenoduodenostomy를 선호하고 있다(recipient procedure 그림 9. 참조). Exocrine drainage는 graft duodenum을 통하여 recipient의 bowel 또는 bladder로 연결되며, ischemic change 또는 rejection으로 leakage가 발생할 수 있다. JP color와 JP amylase, lipase level을 측정하여 monitoring 할 수 있다.

3. Graft survival after pancreas transplantation

- 췌장이식의 성적은 수술 기술의 향상과 더불어 향상되었으나 여전히
  초반 합병증으로 인한 re-laparotomy rate는 30%에 이르는 것으로
  알려져 있다. (Laftavi MR et al., Curr Opin Organ Transplant 2017,
  22(4): 389-397.) 그렇기 때문에 이식 초반 graft failure risk 가 높으며,
  수술 방법 중에서는 SPKT의 성적이 가장 좋은 것으로 알려져 있다.

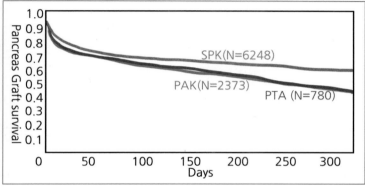

<그림 1. 췌장 이식의 성적은 췌장이식의 종류에 따라 달리 보고되고 있다. 신췌동시이식(SPKT)
이 가장 좋은 성적을 보이고 있다. Axelrod DA et al., Am J Transplant 2010,10(4): 837-845.>

II. Donor management

1. Donor graft quality estimation

1) Pancreas transplantation은 많은 건수가 이루어지지 않기 때문에 간
   또는 신장에 비하여 optimal donor에 대한 연구가 충분히 이루어 지
   지 못하였다.

2) Donor 의 연령, body mass index (BMI), cold ischemic time (CIT)
   는 높을수록 이식 후 성적이 좋지 않다는 것이 보고되었고, 육안소견

상 pancreas graft의 지방침윤, 섬유화 및 석회화 정도가 나쁜 예후와 관련 있다고 보고되었다. (Shapey et al., BMJ 2017, 358: j3784) 하지만 모든 센터가 공유하는 optimal donor selection criteria는 아직 보고되고 있지 않다.

3) SMC donor selection criteria

   (1) Age < 45 years old

   (2) BMI < 30 kg/m^2

   (3) Procurement시 육안상 fat infiltration이 없고 pancreas가 단단하지 않은 경우

CHAPTER 17.

PANCREAS TRANSPLANTATION PROCEDURE

I. Donor procurement procedure

1. Omentectomy 및 pancreas body 확인

1) T-colon과 붙어 있는 greater omentum을 박리하여 lesser sac을 open하고 pancreas body를 노출 시킨다. Pancreas body의 육안소 견을 확인하고 촉지하여 pancreas transplantation의 가능성을 가 늠한다. Duodenum 쪽으로 진행할 때 Rt. Gastro-epiploic vessel을 ligation하고 duodenum 1st and 2nd portion을 적출할 수 있을 정도 로 깨끗하게 정리한다. Omentectomy는 spleen 쪽으로도 진행하여 spleen과 colon을 분리시키고, stomach의 short gastric vessel들도 모 두 ligation하여 spleen과 stomach을 분리시킨다.

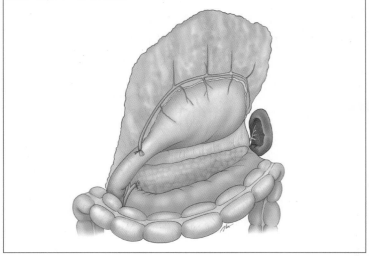

<그림 1. Omentectomy 및 pancreas body 확인>

2) Cocherization 및 pancreas head portion 확인

  (1) Cocherization을 하여 pancreas head를 노출 시키고 촉지하여
단단한 정도를 확인한다. 이때 Lt. renal vein 위쪽으로 주행하
는 superior mesenteric artery (SMA)를 촉지하고 encircling 해
둔다. 이후 duodenum irrigation을 위하여 duodenum은 Treitz
ligament까지 박리하여 가능한 곧게 펴지도록 해준다.

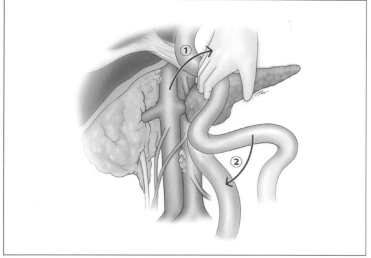

<그림 2. Cocherization 및 pancreas head portion 확인>

3) Pancreas body 박리

(1) Pancreas transplantation을 진행하기로 결정하였다면 spleen을 잡고 들어올려 pancreas의 후면을 retroperitoneal space로부터 박리한다. 이 과정에서 pancreas 손으로 잡지 않고 spleen을 이용하여 manipulation한다. Celiac trunk 의 옆면까지 박리가 가능하다.

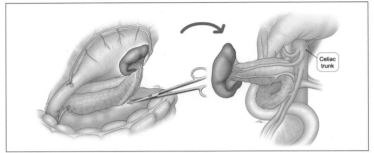

<그림 3. Pancreas body 박리>

4) Duodenum irrigation

　　(1) L-tube를 duodenum 4th portion까지 진입시키고 GIA를 이용하
　　　여 distal과 분리한 뒤 미리 준비해둔 antibiotics solution (NS 500
　　　cc + amphotericin 1V + gentamicin 2A)으로 irrigation 한다.
　　　Irrigation이 끝나면 L-tube를 stomach의 pylorus 상방으로 후퇴시
　　　킨 뒤 pylorus 직하방의 duodenum을 GIA로 분리시킨다.　여기까
　　　지 진행 후 perfusion team에게 수술을 인계한다.

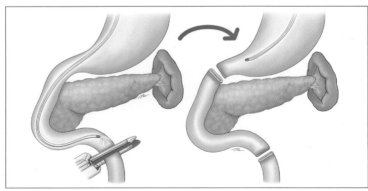

<그림 4. Duodenum irrigation>

5) SMA & SMV trunk 분리

(1) Perfusion이 끝나고 liver graft procurement 시 gastro-duodenal artery와 splenic artery의 위치를 표시하여 잃어버리지 않도록 한다. Portal vein division line은 liver transplantation team과 상의하여 결정한다(보통 Coronary vein level 정도). Liver graft가 나가면 inferior mesenteric vein (IMV)에 cannulation되어 있는 catheter를 제거하고 ligation한다. SMA와 SMV의 trunk는 mesentery와 함께 vascular TA를 사용하여 division한다. 이 때 가능한 pancreas body와 멀게 하여 collateral vessel이 손상되지 않도록 주의한다. 이후 SMA를 aorta에서 잘라내면 pancreas graft가 나오게 된다. SMA와 renal artery의 간격이 좁으므로 renal artery의 손상을 주의해야 한다.

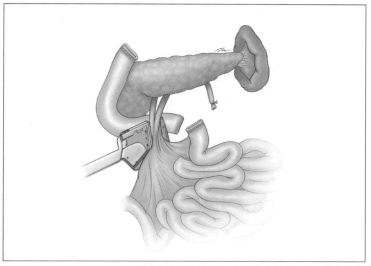

<그림 5. SMA & SMV trunk 분리, IMV를 ligation 해야 한다>

2. Bench procedure

1. Pancreas graft는 duodenum와 pancreas가 en-bloc으로 이식된다. Pancreas와 duodenum은 SMA와 splenic artery 및 gastroduodenal artery (GDA)에서 arterial supply를 받는데, GDA는 SMA와 communication을 이루고 있기 때문에 graft reperfusion 후 back flow가 있는 것을 확인한 후 ligation 한다.

2. SMA와 splenic artery는 donor의 iliac artery Y graft를 이용하여 하나로 만들어 준다. Portal vein은 donor의 iliac vein 또는 IVC graft를 이용하여 elongation 할 수 있지만, 가능한 graft portal vein의 길이를 짧게 하기 위하여 꼭 필요로 하지 않는 경우 그대로 anastomosis를 시행한다.

3. Spleen과 분리하는 부위 및 pancreas 후면의 connective tissue에서 작은 혈관들이 많고 bleeding 하는 경우가 많기 때문에 meticulous ligation을 시행한다.

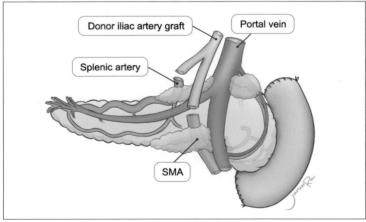

<그림 6. Pancreas graft 의 bench procedure, pancreas graft의 posterior aspect>

II. Recipient procedure

※ Recipient procedure는 KT와의 순서와, exocrine drainage의 방법에 따라 분류될 수 있다.

1. KT와의 순서 관계

1) Spontaneous pancreas kidney transplantation (SPKT)

   - Pancreas와 kidney를 동시에 이식하는 방법으로 kidney graft를 monitoring하여 pancreas rejection을 예측할 수 있다는 장점이 있다.

2) Pancreas transplantation after kidney transplantation (PAK)

   - KT recipient 중 DM을 가지고 있는 환자에게 다른 donor의 pancreas를 이식하는 방법이다. DM으로 인한 end stage renal disease (ESRD) 환자에게 KT를 시행하는 경우 PAK의 가능성을 염두에 두고 왼쪽에 kidney graft를 이식하는 것이 좋다.

3) Pancreas transplantation alone (PTA)

   - DM 환자 중 kidney function이 유지되고 있는 환자에게 pancreas 만을 이식하는 방법이다.

2. Exocrine secretion의 drainage의 방법

1) Bladder drainage

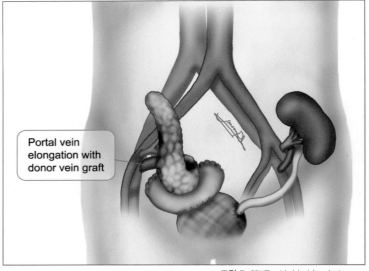

<그림 7. SPKT with bladder drainage>

- 장점 : urine amylase 측정으로 pancreas graft rejection의 monitoring
- 단점 : pancreatic juice (bicarbonate)의 소실로 metabolic acidosis 발생

2) Enteric drainage

(1) Ileal drainage

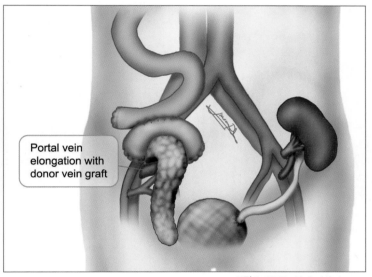

Portal vein elongation with donor vein graft

<그림 8. SPKT with ileal drainage>

- 장점 : bladder drainage로 인한 metabolic acidosis의 문제 해결
- 단점 : small bowel leakage의 위험성 및 portal vein elongation 필요

(2) Duodenal drainage

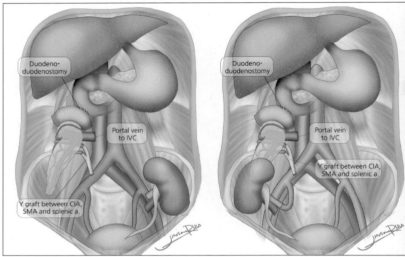

<그림 9. SPKT with duodenal drainage>

- 장점 : bladder drainage로 인한 metabolic acidosis 문제 해결, portal vein elongation을 하지 않을 수 있음. Kidney 와 같은 side 에 이식 가능.
- 단점 : duodenal leakage의 위험성

CHAPTER 18.

PANCREAS TRANSPLANTATION PROTOCOL

〈POSTOP order Pancreas Transplantation Alone or PAK case〉

1. Check V/S q 1hr
2. BR with SFP & Rt. hip flexion and leg elevation
3. NPO except medication
4. Check I/O q 1hr (hourly urine check)
5. Check Bwt
6. CVP monitoring q 4hr
7. Keep Foley in situ
8. Keep L-tube in situ with natural drainage
9. Cough & deep breath q 2hr & incentive spirometer q 1hr while awake
10. Anti-embolic stockings & Vascular Refilling detector until ambulation
11. Check bilateral lower extremity pulses q 1hr

12. Avoid IM injection on right buttock

13. 0.1% chlorhexidine gargling q 6hr

14. 12hr urine collection for Ccr (from 6PM to 6AM)

15. Insulin control

  1) Target BST는 150 (140 ~ 180) mg/dl

  2) Check BST q 1hr ⇨ 2hr ⇨ 4hr (with sustained level)

    : If BGL < 80 or ≥ 250, △BGL > 80 ⇨ recheck 2hrs later

  3) Initiation

    (1) 200 mg/dl < BGL ≤ 250 mg/dl ⇨ starting rate: 1unit/hr

    (2) 250 mg/dl < BGL ⇨ starting rate: 2unit/hr

  4) Maintenance

    (1) BGL < 80 ⇨ RI stop & notify to Dr.

    (2) BGL < 200 ⇨ RI stop

    (3) 200 < BGL ≤ 250 ⇨ 1 unit/hr

    (4) 250 < BGL ≤ 300 ⇨ 2 unit/hr : BST recheck 2hr later

    (5) 300 < BGL ≤ 350 ⇨ 3 unit/hr : BST recheck 2hr later

    (6) 350 < BGL ⇨ 4 unit/hr & notify to Dr.

16. 5% DW half saline 1 L iv c 40 mL/hr

17. 5% albumin 20 mL/hr

18. Hartman solution 60 mL/hr

19. Alprostadil (1.47 ug/kg in NS 50 mL) x2 mivs c 4 cc/hr (총 14번)

20. Gabexate (20 mg/kg in NS 50 mL) mivs c 2 cc/hr (POD#0-6)

21. Heparization nomogram without loading dose (depending on artery state and bleeding tendency)

  - Appendix. Heparin nomogram 참조.

22. Cefotaxime 1.0 g iv q 8hrs (renal function 에 따라 조절하여야 함)

23. Ampicilin/sulbactam 1.5 g 1A q 6hrs

24. Antifungal Prophylaxis

  : Itraconazole syrup 100 mg Q12 (During NPO)

25. Famotidine 1A + NS 50 mL iv q 12hr

26. Ambroxol 1A ivs q 8hr

27. Diogel 1p HS

28. Octreotide 100mcq sc q 8hrs

29. PRN) Nifedipine 10 mg SL (If SBP > 160)

30. PRN) Morphine 2 mg iv

31. CBC, e, chemistry, ion Ca, PT/aPTT, S-osm, ABGA, UA c micro, urine (e, osm), Chest AP (p) amylase/lipase

32. CBC, e, BUN/Cr, S-osm/U-osm q 8hr

33. C-peptide, HbA1C, Proinsulin/insulin : twice a week

34. MPA level : twice a week until postOp 2 wks

35. Immunosuppression

: rATG induction (1.5 mg/kg) + 5 dw 250 mL IVS over 10 hour

1) MPD 500 mg ivs q 24hr

2) ganciclovir 2.5 mg/kg + NS 50 cc ivs q 12 hrs (Prophylaxis) : renal function 에 따라 조절

3) SMX-TMP 1T po WM

4) Acetaminophen 125 mg 5T (rATG 투여 전)

5) Chlorpheniramine 1A ivs (rATG 투여 전)

36. POD#1,3,5 Doppler Sono of pancreas

* Immune suppression

1. rATG 1.5 mg/kg

2. 2일째부터 Tacrolimus를 overlap.

3. Check Tacrolimus level

⟨ PAK POD #1 day ⟩

1. Check V/S q 1hr
2. BR with SFP & Rt. Hip flexion and leg elevation
3. NPO except for medication
4. Check I/O q 1hr (hourly urine check)
5. Check Bwt
6. CVP monitoring q 4hr
7. Keep Foley in situ
8. Keep L-tube in situ with natural drainage
9. Cough & deep breath q 2hr & incentive spirometer q 1hr while awake
10. Anti-embolic stockings & Vascular refilling detector until ambulation
11. Check bilateral lower extremity pulses q 1hr
12. Avoid IM injection on right buttock
13. 0.1% chlorhexidine gargling q 6hr
14. 24hr urine collection for Ccr (from 6 AM to 6 AM)
15. Insulin control
   1) Target BST ≒ 150 (140 ~ 180) mg/dl
   2) Check BST q 1hr ⇨ 2hr ⇨ 4hr (with sustained level)
      : If BGL < 80 or ≥ 250, △BGL > 80 ⇨ recheck 2hrs later
   3) Initiation
      (1) 200 mg/dl < BGL ≤ 250 mg/dl ⇨ starting rate: 1unit/hr
      (2) 250 mg/dl < BGL ⇨ starting rate: 2unit/hr
   4) Maintenance
      (1) BGL < 80 ⇨ RI stop & notify to Dr.
      (2) BGL < 200 ⇨ RI stop
      (3) 200 < BGL ≤ 250 ⇨ 1 unit/hr
      (4) 250 < BGL ≤ 300 ⇨ 2 unit/hr : BST recheck 2hr later
      (5) 300 < BGL ≤ 350 ⇨ 3 unit/hr : BST recheck 2hr later
      (6) 350 < BGL ⇨ 4 unit/hr & notify to Dr.
16. 5% DW half saline 1 L iv c 40 mL/hr
17. 5% albumin 20 mL/hr

18. Hartman solution 1 L 20 mL/hr
19. Combiflex peri 1100 1.1 L c 40 mL/hr : 12%미만
20. Alprostadil   (1.47 ug/kg in NS 50 mL) x2 mivs c 4 cc/hr
21. Gabexate   (20 mg/kg in NS 50 mL) mivs c 2 cc/hr
22. Heparization nomogram without loading dose (depending on artery state and bleeding tendency)
23. Cefotaxime 2 g iv q 8 hrs (renal function 에 따라 조절하여야 함)
24. Ampicillin/Sulbactam 1.5 g q 6hrs
25. Antifungal Prophylaxis
  Itraconazole syrup 100 mg q12
26. Famotidine 1A + NS 50 mL iv q 12hr
27. Ambroxol 1A ivs q 8hr
28. Diogel 1p PLT HS
29. Octreotide 100 mcg sc q 8 hr
30. PRN) Nifedipine 10 mg SL (If SBP > 160)
31. PRN) Morphine 2 mg iv
32. CBC, e, chemistry, ion Ca, PT/aPTT, S-osm, ABGA, VBGA (Bladder drainage 시), UA c micro, urine (e, osm, amylase (Bladder drainage 시)), chest AP (portable) amylase/lipase
33. CBC, e, BUN/Cr, S-osm/U-osm q 8hr
34. C-peptide, HbA1C, Proinsulin/insulin : twice per week
35. POD#1,3,5 Doppler Sono of pancreas & kidney
  POD#2,7 contrast CT (renal function 및 수술 당시 vessel 상태에 따라 고려)
36. Immunosuppression
  1) rATG 1.5 mg/kg + 5 dw 250 mL ivs over 2hr
  2) MPD 125 mg ivs q 24hr
  3) ganciclovir 2.5 mg/kg + NS 50 cc ivs q 12 hrs (Prophylaxis) :
    renal function에 따라 조절
  4) SMX-TMP 1T po WM
  5) Acetaminophen 125 mg 5T (rATG 투여 전)
  6) Chlorpheniramine 1A ivs (rATG 투여 전)

⟨ PAK POD #2 ⟩

1. Check V/S q 1hr
2. BR with SFP & Rt. hip flexion and leg elevation
3. NPO except medication
4. Check I/O q 1hr (hourly urine check)
5. Check Bwt
6. CVP monitoring q 4hr
7. Keep Foley in situ with natural drainage
8. Keep L-tube in situ
9. Cough & deep breath q 2hr & incentive spirometer q 1hr while awake
10. Anti-embolic stockings & Vascular refilling detector until ambulation
11. Check bilateral lower extremity pulses q 1hr
12. Avoid IM injection on right buttock
13. 0.1 chlorhexidine gargling q 6hr
14. 24hr urine collection for Ccr (from 6AM to 6AM)
15. Insulin control
   1) Target BST ≒ 150 (140 ~ 180) mg/dl
   2) Check BST q 1hr ⇨ 2hr ⇨ 4hr (with sustained level)
      : If BGL < 80 or ≥ 250, △BGL > 80 ⇨ recheck 2hrs later
   3) Initiation
      (1) 200 mg/dl < BGL ≤ 250 mg/dl ⇨ starting rate: 1unit/hr
      (2) 250 mg/dl < BGL ⇨ starting rate: 2unit/hr
   4) Maintenance
      (1) BGL < 80 ⇨ RI stop & notify to Dr.
      (2) BGL < 200 ⇨ RI stop
      (3) 200 < BGL ≤ 250 ⇨ 1 unit/hr
      (4) 250 < BGL ≤ 300 ⇨ 2 unit/hr : BST recheck 2hr later
      (5) 300 < BGL ≤ 350 ⇨ 3 unit/hr : BST recheck 2hr later
      (6) 350 < BGL ⇨ 4 unit/hr & notify to Dr.

16. 5% DW half saline iv c 40 mL/hr

17. Combiflex peri 1100 1.1 L c 40 mL/hr

18. 5% albumin 20 mL/hr

19. Hartman 1 L 20 mL/hr

20. Alprostadil   (1.47 ug/kg in NS 50 mL) x2 mivs c 4cc/hr

21. Gabexate   (20 mg/kg in NS 50 mL) mivs c 2cc/hr

22. Heparization nomogram without loading dose (depending on artery state and bleeding tendency)

23. Cefotaxime 2 g iv q 8hrs (renal function 에 따라 조절하여야 함)

24. Ampicillin / Sulbactam 1.5 g q 6hrs

25. Itraconazole 100 mg PLT Q12

26. Famotidine 1A + NS 50 mL iv q 12hr

27. Diogel 1p PLT HS

28. Octreotide 100 mcg sc q 8 hr

29. Ambroxol 1A ivs q 8hr

30. PRN) Nifedipine 10 mg SL (If SBP > 160)

31. PRN) Morphine 2 mg iv

32. CBC, e, chemistry, ion Ca, PT/aPTT, S-osm, ABGA, VBGA (Bladder drainage 시), UA c micro, urine (e, osm, amylase (Bladder drainage 시)), chest AP (portable) amylase/lipase

33. CBC, e, BUN/Cr, S-osm/U-osm q 8hr

34. C-peptide, HbA1C, Proinsulin/insulin : twice a week

35. Tacrolimus / MMF po start

36. Immunosuppression

  1) rATG 1.5 mg/kg + 5 dw 250 mL ivs over 2hr

  2) MPD 125 mg ivs q 24hr

  3) Ganciclovir 2.5 mg/kg + NS 50 cc ivs q 12 hrs (Prophylaxis) : renal function에 따라 조절

  4) SMX-TMP 1T po WM

  5) Acetaminophen 125 mg 5T (rATG 투여 전)

  6) Chlorpheniramine 1A ivs (rATG 투여 전)

〈 PAK POD #3 〉

1. Check V/S q 1hr
2. BR with SFP & Rt. Hip flexion and leg elevation
3. NPO except for medication : POD#5까지
4. Check I/O q 8hr (hourly urine check)
5. Check Bwt
6. CVP monitoring q 4hr
7. Keep Foley in situ
8. Bowel movement에 따라 L-tube remove 고려
9. Cough & deep breath q 2hr & incentive spirometer q 1hr while awake
10. Anti-embolic stockings & Vascular refilling detector until ambulation
11. Check bilateral lower extremity pulses q 1hr
12. Avoid IM injection on right buttock
13. 0.1 % chlorhexidine gargling q 6hr
14. 24hr urine collection for Ccr (from 6 AM to 6 AM)
15. Insulin control

  1) Target BST는 150 (140 ~ 180) mg/dl

  2) Check BST q 1hr ⇨ 2hr ⇨ 4hr (with sustained level)

     : If BGL < 80 or ≥ 250, △BGL > 80 ⇨ recheck 2hrs later

  3) Initiation

     (1) 200 mg/dl < BGL ≤ 250 mg/dl ⇨ starting rate: 1unit/hr

     (2) 250 mg/dl < BGL ⇨ starting rate: 2unit/hr

  4) Maintenance

     (1) BGL < 80 ⇨ RI stop & notify to Dr.

     (2) BGL < 200 ⇨ RI stop

     (3) 200 < BGL ≤ 250 ⇨ 1 unit/hr

     (4) 250 < BGL ≤ 300 ⇨ 2 unit/hr : BST recheck 2hr later

     (5) 300 < BGL ≤ 350 ⇨ 3 unit/hr : BST recheck 2hr later

     (6) 350 < BGL ⇨ 4 unit/hr & notify to Dr.

16. 5% DW half saline iv c 40 mL/hr
17. Combiflex peri 1100 1.1 L c 40 mL/hr
18. 5% albumin 20 mL/hr
19. Hartman 1 L 20 mL/hr
20. Alprostadil   (1.47 ug/kg in NS 50 mL) x2 mivs c 4 cc/hr
21. Gabexate   (20 mg/kg in NS 50 mL) mivs c 2 cc/hr
22. Heparization nomogram without loading dose (depending on artery state and bleeding tendency)
23. Cefotaxime 2 g iv q 8hrs (renal function에 따라 조절하여야 함)
24. Ampicillin/sulbactam 1.5 g q 6hrs
25. Itraconazole syrup 100 mg Q12
26. Famotidine 1A + NS 50 mL iv q 12hr
27. Diogel 1p HS
28. Octreotide 100 mcg sc q 8 hr
29. Ambroxol 1A ivs q 8hr
30. PRN) Nifedipine 10 mg SL (If SBP > 160)
31. PRN) Morphine 2 mg iv
32. CBC, e, chemistry, ion Ca, PT/aPTT, S-osm, ABGA, VBGA (Bladder drainage 시), UA c micro, urine (e, osm, amylase (Bladder drainage 시)), chest AP (portable) amylase/lipase
33. CBC, e, BUN/Cr, S-osm/U-osm q 8hr
34. C-peptide, HbA1C, Proinsulin/insulin : twice a week
35. Immunosuppression
36. POD#1,3,5 Doppler Sono of pancreas

〈 PAK POD #4 〉

1. Check V/S q 1hr
2. BR with SFP & Rt. hip flexion and leg elevation
3. NPO except medication : POD#5까지
4. Check I/O q 1hr (hourly urine check)
5. Check Bwt
6. CVP monitoring q 4hr
7. Keep Foley in situ
8. Cough & deep breath q 2hr & incentive spirometer q 1hr while awake
9. Anti-embolic stockings & Vascular refilling detector until ambulation
10. Check bilateral lower extremity pulses q 1hr
11. Avoid IM injection on right buttock
12. 0.1% chlorhexidine gargling q 6hr
13. 24hr urine collection for Ccr (from 6AM to 6AM)
14. Insulin control
    1) Target BST는 150 (140 ~ 180) mg/dl
    2) Check BST q 1hr ⇨ 2hr ⇨ 4hr (with sustained level)
       : If BGL < 80 or ≥ 250, △BGL > 80 ⇨ recheck 2hrs later
    3) Initiation
       (1) 200 mg/dl < BGL ≤ 250 mg/dl ⇨ starting rate: 1unit/hr
       (2) 250 mg/dl < BGL ⇨ starting rate: 2unit/hr
    4) Maintenance
       (1) BGL < 80 ⇨ RI stop & notify to Dr.
       (2) BGL < 200 ⇨ RI stop
       (3) 200 < BGL ≤ 250 ⇨ 1 unit/hr
       (4) 250 < BGL ≤ 300 ⇨ 2 unit/hr : BST recheck 2hr later
       (5) 300 < BGL ≤ 350 ⇨ 3 unit/hr : BST recheck 2hr later
       (6) 350 < BGL ⇨ 4 unit/hr & notify to Dr.
15. 5% DW half saline iv c 40 mL/hr

16. Combiflex peri 1100 1.1 L c 40mL/hr
17. Half saline 1 L : 20 mL/hr
18. Hour Urine < 50 mL → call Dr
19. 5% albumin 20 mL/hr
20. Alprostadil   (1.47 ug/kg in NS 50 mL) x2 mivs c 4 cc/hr
21. Gabexate   (20 mg/kg in NS 50 mL) mivs c 2 cc/hr
22. Heparization nomogram without loading dose (depending on artery state and bleeding tendency)
23. Cefotaxime 2 g iv q 8hrs (renal function 에 따라 조절하여야 함)
24. Ampicillin/sulbactam 1.5 g q 6hrs
25. Itraconazole syrup 100 mg PLT Q12
26. Famotidine 1A + NS 50 mL iv q 12hr
27. Diogel 1p PLT HS
28. Octreotide 100 mcg sc q 8 hr
29. Ambroxol 1A ivs q 8hr
30. PRN) Nifedipine 10 mg SL (If SBP > 160)
31. PRN) Morphine 2 mg iv
32. CBC, e, chemistry, ion Ca, PT/aPTT, S-osm, ABGA, VBGA (Bladder drainage 시), UA c micro, urine (e, osm, amylase (Bladder drainage 시)), chest AP (portable) amylase/lipase
33. CBC, e, BUN/Cr, S-osm/U-osm q 8hr
34. C-peptide, HbA1C, Proinsulin/insulin : Twice a week
35. Immunosuppression

〈 PAK POD #5 〉

1. Check V/S q 1hr
2. BR with SFP & Rt. Hip flexion and leg elevation
3. Sips of water: 천천히 diet 진행
4. Check I/O q 1hr (hourly urine check)
5. Check Bwt
6. CVP monltoring q 4hr
7. Keep Foley in situ
8. Cough & deep breath q 2hr
9. Anti-embolic stockings & Vascular refilling detector until ambulation
10. Check bilateral lower extremity pulses q 1hr
11. Avoid IM injection on right buttock
12. 0.1% chlorhexidine gargling q 6hr
13. 24hr urine collection for Ccr (from 6 AM to 6 AM)
14. Insulin control
    1) Target BST는 150 (140 ~ 180) mg/dl
    2) Check BST q 1hr ⇨ 2hr ⇨ 4hr (with sustained level)
       : If BGL < 80 or ≥ 250, △BGL > 80 ⇨ recheck 2hrs later
    3) Initiation
       (1) 200 mg/dl < BGL ≤ 250 mg/dl ⇨ starting rate: 1unit/hr
       (2) 250 mg/dl < BGL ⇨ starting rate: 2unit/hr
    4) Maintenance
       (1) BGL < 80 ⇨ RI stop & notify to Dr.
       (2) BGL < 200 ⇨ RI stop
       (3) 200 < BGL ≤ 250 ⇨ 1 unit/hr
       (4) 250 < BGL ≤ 300 ⇨ 2 unit/hr : BST recheck 2hr later
       (5) 300 < BGL ≤ 350 ⇨ 3 unit/hr : BST recheck 2hr later
       (6) 350 < BGL ⇨ 4 unit/hr & notify to Dr.
15. 5% DW half saline iv c 40 mL/hr
16. Combiflex peri 1100 1.1 L c 40 mL/hr

17. 5% albumin 20 mL/hr
18. Alprostadil   (1.47 ug/kg in NS 50 mL) x2 mivs c 4 cc/hr
19. Gabexate   (20 mg/kg in NS 50 mL) mivs c 2 cc/hr
20. Heparization nomogram without loading dose (depending on artery state and bleeding tendency)
21. Cefotaxime 2 g iv q 8hrs (renal function 에 따라 조절하여야 함)
22. Ampicillin/sulbactam 1.5 g q 6hrs
23. Itraconazole syrup 100 mg PLT bid
24. Consider Clopidogrel, Warfarin (POD #5 start)
25. Famotidine 1A + NS 50 mL iv q 12hr
26. Diogel 1p PLT HS
27. Octreotide 100 mcg sc q 8 hr
28. Ambroxol 1A ivs q 8hr
29. PRN) Nifedipine 10 mg SL (If SBP > 160)
30. PRN) Morphine 2 mg iv
31. CBC, e, chemistry, ion Ca, PT/aPTT, S-osm, ABGA, VBGA (Bladder drainage 시), UA c micro, urine (e, osm, amylase (Bladder drainage 시)), chest AP (portable) amylase/lipase
32. CBC, e, BUN/Cr, S-osm/U-osm q 8hr
33. C-peptide, HbA1C, Proinsulin/insulin : twice a week
34. Immunosuppression
35. POD#1,3,5 Doppler Sono of pancreas
36. POD#2,7 contrast CT (renal function에 따라)
37. Foley remove after checking DTPA and CT angiography
    J-P remove when patient is stable after enough diet
38. Move to general ward depending on patient condition
39. Consult to Infectionist part before discharge and make an appoint at Out patient department
40. CMV 및 bacterial 검사는 kidney transplantation patient에 준하여 검사한다.
    치료 역시 kidney transplantation 환자에 준하여 시행

⟨ POSTOP order SPK case ⟩

1. Check V/S q 1hr
2. BR with SFP & Rt. Hip flexion and leg elevation
3. NPO except for medication
4. Check I/O q 1hr
5. Check Bwt
6. CVP monitoring q 4hr
7. Keep Foley in situ
8. Keep L-tube in situ with natural drainage
9. Cough & deep breath q 2hr & incentive spirometer q 1hr while awake
10. Anti-embolic stockings & Vascular Refilling detector until ambulation
11. Check bilateral lower extremity pulses q 1hr
12. Avoid IM injection on right buttock
13. 0. 1% chlorhexidine gargling q 6hr
14. 12hr urine collection for Ccr (from 6 PM to 6 AM)
15. Insulin control
    1) Target BST늘 150 (140 ~ 180) mg/dl
    2) Check BST q 1hr ⇨ 2hr ⇨ 4hr (with sustained level)
       : If BGL < 80 or ≥ 250, △BGL > 80 ⇨ recheck 2hrs later
    3) Initiation
       (1) 200 mg/dl < BGL ≤ 250 mg/dl ⇨ starting rate: 1unit/hr
       (2) 250 mg/dl < BGL ⇨ starting rate: 2unit/hr
    4) Maintenance
       (1) BGL < 80 ⇨ RI stop & notify to Dr.
       (2) BGL < 200 ⇨ RI stop
       (3) 200 < BGL ≤ 250 ⇨ 1 unit/hr
       (4) 250 < BGL ≤ 300 ⇨ 2 unit/hr : BST recheck 2hr later
       (5) 300 < BGL ≤ 350 ⇨ 3 unit/hr : BST recheck 2hr later
       (6) 350 < BGL ⇨ 4 unit/hr & notify to Dr.

16. 5% DW half saline iv c 40 mL/hr
17. Post transplantation solution(Half saline 1 L) replace

    H/U   <50 mL → call Dr.

    50-100 mL → 150%

    100-200 mL → 120%

    200-300 mL → 100%

    300-500 mL → 80%

    >500 mL → 60%

    CVP replacement with Volulyte.

    If CVP < 4 mmHg ⇨ 2 cc/kg/hr ⇨ recheck 2hr later

    < 10 mmHg ⇨ 1 cc/kg/hr

    10-12 mmHg ⇨ stop

18. Alprostadil (1.47 ug/kg in NS 50 mL) x2 mivs c 4 cc/hr (총 14번 투여)
19. Gabexate (20 mg/kg in NS 50 mL) mivs c 2 cc/hr (POD#0-6)
20. Heparization nomogram without loading dose (depending on artery state and bleeding tendency)

   - Appendix. Heparin nomogram 참조
21. Cefotaxime 2.0 g iv q 8hrs (renal function 에 따라 조절하여야 함)
22. Ampicillin/sulbactam 1.5 g q 6hrs
23. Antifungal Prophylaxis

    : Itraconazole syrup 100 mg bid PLT (During NPO)
24. Famotidine 1A + NS 50 mL iv q 12hr
25. Ambroxol 1A ivs q 8hr
26. Diogel 1p PLT HS
27. Octreotide 100 mcg sc q 8 hr
28. PRN) Nifedipine 10 mg SL (If SBP > 160)
29. PRN) Morphine 2 mg iv
30. CBC, e, chemistry, ion Ca, PT/aPTT, S-osm, ABGA, UA c micro, urine (e, osm), Chest AP (p) amylase/lipase

31. CBC, e, BUN/Cr, S-osm/U-osm q 8hr
32. C-peptide, HbA1C, Proinsulin/insulin : twice a week
33. Immunosuppression
    : rATG based induction & Triple Drug based maintenance
34. POD#1,3,5 Doppler Sono of pancreas & kidney

〈 SPK POD #1 〉

1. Check V/S q 1hr
2. BR with SFP & Rt. Hip flexion and leg elevation
3. NPO except for medication
4. Check I/O q 1hr
5. Check Bwt
6. CVP monitoring q 4hr
7. Keep Foley in situ
8. Keep L-tube in situ with natural drainage
9. Cough & deep breath q 2hr & incentive spirometer q 1hr while awake
10. Anti-embolic stockings & Vascular refilling detector until ambulation
11. Check bilateral lower extremity pulses q 1hr
12. Avoid IM injection on right buttock
13. 0.1% chlorhexidine gargling q 6hr
14. 24hr urine collection for Ccr (from 6 AM to 6 AM)
15. Insulin control

   1) Target BST≒150 (140 ~ 180) mg/dl
   2) Check BST q 1hr ⇨ 2hr ⇨ 4hr (with sustained level)

      : If BGL < 80 or ≥ 250, △BGL > 80 ⇨ recheck 2hrs later

   3) Initiation

      (1) 200 mg/dl < BGL ≤ 250 mg/dl ⇨ starting rate: 1unit/hr
      (2) 250 mg/dl < BGL ⇨ starting rate: 2unit/hr

   4) Maintenance

      (1) BGL < 80 ⇨ RI stop & notify to Dr.
      (2) BGL < 200 ⇨ RI stop
      (3) 200 < BGL ≤ 250 ⇨ 1 unit/hr
      (4) 250 < BGL ≤ 300 ⇨ 2 unit/hr : BST recheck 2hr later
      (5) 300 < BGL ≤ 350 ⇨ 3 unit/hr : BST recheck 2hr later
      (6) 350 < BGL ⇨ 4 unit/hr & notify to Dr.

16. 5% DW half saline iv c 40 mL/hr
17. Post transplantation solution (Half saline 1 L) replace

   H/U   <50 mL → call Dr.

   50-100 mL → 120%

   100-200 mL → 100%

   200-300 mL → 80%

   300-500 mL → 60%

   >500 mL → 50%

   CVP replacement with Volulyte.

   If CVP < 4 mmHg ⇨ 2 cc/kg/hr ⇨ recheck 2hr later

   < 10 mmHg ⇨ 1 cc/kg/hr

   10-12 mmHg ⇨ stop
18. Alprostadil   (1.47 ug/kg in NS 50 mL) x2 mivs c 4 cc/hr (총 14회 투여)
19. Gabexate   (20 mg/kg in NS 50 mL) mivs c 2 cc/hr
20. Heparization nomogram without loading dose (depending on artery state and bleeding tendency)
21. Cefotaxime 2 g iv q 8hrs (renal function 에 따라 조절하여야 함)
22. Ampicillin/sulbactam 1.5 g q 6hrs
23. Antifungal Prophylaxis

   Itraconazole syrup 100 mg Q12 PLT
24. Octreotide 100q sc q 8 hr
25. Famotidine 1A + NS 50mL iv q 12hr
26. Ambroxol 1A q 8 hr
27. Diogel 1p PLT HS
28. PRN) Nifedipine 10 mg SL (If SBP > 160)
29. PRN) Morphine 2 mg iv
30. CBC, e, chemistry, ion Ca, PT/aPTT, S-osm, ABGA, UA c micro, urine (e, osm), chest AP (portable) amylase/lipase
31. CBC, e, BUN/Cr, S-osm/U-osm q 8 hr

32. C-peptide, HbA1C, Proinsulin/insulin : Twice a week
33. POD#1,3,5- Doppler Sono of pancreas & kidney
34. Immunosuppression

〈 SPK POD #2 〉

1. Check V/S q 1hr
2. BR with SFP & Rt. Hip flexion and leg elevation
3. NPO except for medication
4. Check I/O q 1hr
5. Check Bwt
6. CVP monitoring q 4hr
7. Keep Foley in situ
8. Keep L-tube in situ with natural drainage
9. Cough & deep breath q 2hr & incentive spirometer q 1hr while awake
10. Anti-embolic stockings & Vascular refilling detector until ambulation
11. Check bilateral lower extremity pulses q 1hr
12. Avoid IM injection on right buttock
13. 0.1% chlorhexidine gargling q 6hr
14. 24hr urine collection for Ccr (from 6 AM to 6 AM)
15. Insulin control
   1) Target BST는 150 (140 ~ 180) mg/dl
   2) Check BST q 1hr ⇨ 2hr ⇨ 4hr (with sustained level)
      : If BGL < 80 or ≥ 250, △BGL > 80 ⇨ recheck 2hrs later
   3) Initiation
      (1) 200 mg/dl < BGL ≤ 250 mg/dl ⇨ starting rate: 1unit/hr
      (2) 250 mg/dl < BGL ⇨ starting rate: 2unit/hr
   4) Maintenance
      (1) BGL < 80 ⇨ RI stop & notify to Dr.
      (2) BGL < 200 ⇨ RI stop
      (3) 200 < BGL ≤ 250 ⇨ 1 unit/hr
      (4) 250 < BGL ≤ 300 ⇨ 2 unit/hr : BST recheck 2hr later
      (5) 300 < BGL ≤ 350 ⇨ 3 unit/hr : BST recheck 2hr later
      (6) 350 < BGL ⇨ 4 unit/hr & notify to Dr.

16. 5% DW half saline iv c 40 mL/hr
17. Post transplantation solution (Half saline 1 L) replace

    H/U   <50 mL → call Dr.

    50-100 mL → 120%

    100-200 mL → 100%

    200-300 mL → 80%

    300-500 mL → 60%

    >500 mL → 50%

    CVP replacement with Volulyte.

    If CVP < 4 mmHg ⇨ 2 cc/kg/hr ⇨ recheck 2hr later

    < 10 mmHg ⇨ 1 cc/kg/hr

    10-12 mmHg ⇨ stop
18. Alprostadil   (1.47 ug/kg in NS 50mL) x2 mivs c 4 cc/hr (총 14회 투여)
19. Gabexate   (20 mg/kg in NS 50mL) mivs c 2 cc/hr
20. Heparization nomogram without loading dose (depending on artery state and bleeding tendency)
21. Cefotaxime 2 g iv q 8hrs (renal function 에 따라 조절하여야 함)
22. Ampicillin/sulbactam 1.5 g q 6hrs
23. Antifungal Prophylaxis

    Itraconazole syrup 100 mg Q12 PLT
24. Octreotide 100q sc q 8 hr
25. Famotidine 1A + NS 50 mL iv q 12hr
26. Ambroxol 1A q 8 hr
27. Diogel 1p PLT HS
28. PRN) Nifedipine 10 mg SL (If SBP > 160)
29. PRN) Morphine 2 mg iv
30. CBC, e, chemistry, ion Ca, PT/aPTT, S-osm, ABGA, UA c micro, urine (e, osm), chest AP (portable) amylase/lipase
31. CBC, e, BUN/Cr, S-osm/U-osm q 8hr

32. C-peptide, HbA1C, Proinsulin/insulin : Twice a week
33. POD#1,3,5-Doppler Sono of pancreas & kidney
    POD#2,7 contrast CT (renal function에 따라 시행)
34. Immunosuppression

〈 SPK POD #3 〉

1. Check V/S q 1hr
2. BR with SFP & Rt. Hip flexion and leg elevation
3. NPO except for medication : POD#5까지
4. Check I/O q 8hr
5. Bwt check
6. CVP monitoring q 4hr
7. Keep Foley in situ
8. Keep L-tube in situ with natural drainage
9. Cough & deep breath q 2hr & incentive spirometer q 1hr while awake
10. Anti-embolic stockings & Vascular refilling detector until ambulation
11. Check bilateral lower extremity pulses q 1hr
12. Avoid IM injection on right buttock
13. 0.1% chlorhexidine gargling q 6hr
14. 24hr urine collection for Ccr (from 6 AM to 6 AM)
15. Insulin control

   1) Target BST는150 (140 ~ 180) mg/dl

   2) Check BST q 1hr ⇨ 2hr ⇨ 4hr (with sustained level)

      : If BGL < 80 or ≥ 250, △BGL > 80 ⇨ recheck 2hrs later

   3) Initiation

      (1) 200 mg/dl < BGL ≤ 250 mg/dl ⇨ starting rate: 1unit/hr

      (2) 250 mg/dl < BGL ⇨ starting rate: 2unit/hr

   4) Maintenance

      (1) BGL < 80 ⇨ RI stop & notify to Dr.

      (2) BGL < 200 ⇨ RI stop

      (3) 200 < BGL ≤ 250 ⇨ 1 unit/hr

      (4) 250 < BGL ≤ 300 ⇨ 2 unit/hr : BST recheck 2hr later

      (5) 300 < BGL ≤ 350 ⇨ 3 unit/hr : BST recheck 2hr later

      (6) 350 < BGL ⇨ 4 unit/hr & notify to Dr.

16. 5% dextrose half saline + Half saline 1 L iv c 40 mL/hr

17. Combiflex peri 1100 1.1 L c 40 mL/hr

18. Post transplantation solution (Half saline 1 L) replace

    H/U   <50 mL → call Dr.

    50-100 mL → 80%

    100-200 mL → 60%

    200-300 mL → 40%

    300-500 mL → 20%

    >500 mL → 0 %

19. Alprostadil   (1.47 ug/kg in NS 50 mL) x 2 mivs c 4cc/hr

20. Gabexate   (20 mg/kg in NS 50 mL) mivs c 2cc/hr

21. Heparization nomogram without loading dose (depending on artery state and bleeding tendency)

22. Cefotaxime 2 g iv q 8hrs (renal function 에 따라 조절하여야 함)

23. Ampicillin/sulbactam 1.5 g q 6hrs

24. Itraconazole syrup 100 mg PLT Q12

25. Famotidine 1A + NS 50 mL iv q 12hr

26. Ambroxol 1A q 8 hr

27. Diogel 1p PLT HS

28. Octreotide 100q sc q 8 hr

29. PRN) Nifedipine 10 mg SL (If SBP > 160)

30. PRN) Morphine 2 mg iv

31. CBC, e, chemistry, ion Ca, PT/aPTT, S-osm, ABGA, UA c micro, urine (e, osm), chest AP (p) amylase/lipase

32. CBC, e, BUN/Cr, S-osm/U-osm q 8hr

33. C-peptide, HbA1C, Proinsulin/insulin : twice a week

34. Immunosuppression

35. POD#1,3,5 Doppler Sono of pancreas and kidney

〈 SPK POD #4 〉

1. Check V/S q 1hr
2. BR with SFP & Rt. Hip flexion and leg elevation
3. NPO except for medication : POD#5까지
4. Check I/O q 8hr
5. Bwt check
6. CVP monitoring q 4hr
7. Keep Foley in situ
8. Keep L-tube in situ with natural drainage
9. Cough & deep breath q 2hr & incentive spirometer q 1hr while awake
10. Anti-embolic stockings & Vascular refilling detector until ambulation
11. Check bilateral lower extremity pulses q 1hr
12. Avoid IM injection on right buttock
13. 0.1% chlorhexidine gargling q 6hr
14. 24hr urine collection for Ccr (from 6 AM to 6 AM)
15. Insulin control

  1) Target BST는 150 (140 ~ 180) mg/dl

  2) Check BST q 1hr ⇨ 2hr ⇨ 4hr (with sustained level)

   : If BGL < 80 or ≥ 250, △BGL > 80 ⇨ recheck 2hrs later

  3) Initiation

   (1) 200 mg/dl < BGL ≤ 250 mg/dl ⇨ starting rate: 1unit/hr

   (2) 250 mg/dl < BGL ⇨ starting rate: 2unit/hr

  4) Maintenance

   (1) BGL < 80 ⇨ RI stop & notify to Dr.

   (2) BGL < 200 ⇨ RI stop

   (3) 200 < BGL ≤ 250 ⇨ 1 unit/hr

   (4) 250 < BGL ≤ 300 ⇨ 2 unit/hr : BST recheck 2hr later

   (5) 300 < BGL ≤ 350 ⇨ 3 unit/hr : BST recheck 2hr later

   (6) 350 < BGL ⇨ 4 unit/hr & notify to Dr.

16. 5% dextrose half saline + Half saline 1 L iv c 40 mL/hr

17. Combiflex peri 1100 1.1 L c 40 mL/hr

18. Post transplantation solution (Half saline 1 L) replace

    H/U   <50 mL → call Dr.

    50-100 mL → 80%

    100-200 mL → 60%

    200-300 mL → 40%

    300-500 mL → 20%

    >500 mL → 0 %

19. Alprostadil   (1.47 ug/kg in NS 50 mL) x 2 mivs c 4 cc/hr

20. Gabexate   (20 mg/kg in NS 50 mL) mivs c 2 cc/hr

21. Heparization nomogram without loading dose (depending on artery state and bleeding tendency)

22. Cefotaxime 2 g iv q 8hrs (renal function 에 따라 조절하여야 함)

23. Ampicillin/sulbactam 1.5 g q 6hrs

24. Itraconazole syrup 100 mg PLT Q12

25. Famotidine 1A + NS 50 mL iv q 12hr

26. Ambroxol 1A q 8 hr

27. Diogel 1p PLT HS

28. Octreotide 100q sc q 8 hr

29. PRN) Nifedipine 10 mg SL (If SBP > 160)

30. PRN) Morphine 2 mg iv

31. CBC, e, chemistry, ion Ca, PT/aPTT, S-osm, ABGA, UA c micro, urine (e, osm), chest AP (p) amylase/lipase

32. CBC, e, BUN/Cr, S-osm/U-osm q 8hr

33. C-peptide, HbA1C, Proinsulin/insulin : twice a week

34. Immunosuppression

35. POD#1,3,5 Doppler Sono of pancreas and kidney

⟨ SPK POD #5 ⟩

1. Check V/S q 1hr
2. BR with SFP & Rt. Hip flexion and leg elevation
3. Sips of water: 천천히 diet 진행
4. Check I/O q 8hr
5. Bwt check
6. CVP monitoring q 4hr
7. Keep Foley in situ
8. Keep L-tube in situ with natural drainage
9. Cough & deep breath q 2hr
10. Anti-embolic stockings & Vascular refilling detector until ambulation
11. Check bilateral lower extremity pulses q 1hr
12. Avoid IM injection on right buttock
13. 0.1% Chlorhexidine gargling q 6hr
14. 24hr urine collection for Ccr (from 6 AM to 6 AM)
15. Insulin control

 1) Target BST는150 (140 ~ 180) mg/dl
 2) Check BST q 1hr ⇨ 2hr ⇨ 4hr (with sustained level)
   : If BGL < 80 or ≥ 250, △BGL > 80 ⇨ recheck 2hrs later
 3) Initiation
   (1) 200 mg/dl < BGL ≤ 250 mg/dl ⇨ starting rate: 1unit/hr
   (2) 250 mg/dl < BGL ⇨ starting rate: 2unit/hr
 4) Maintenance
   (1) BGL < 80 ⇨ RI stop & notify to Dr.
   (2) BGL < 200 ⇨ RI stop
   (3) 200 < BGL ≤ 250 ⇨ 1 unit/hr
   (4) 250 < BGL ≤ 300 ⇨ 2 unit/hr : BST recheck 2hr later
   (5) 300 < BGL ≤ 350 ⇨ 3 unit/hr : BST recheck 2hr later
   (6) 350 < BGL ⇨ 4 unit/hr & notify to Dr.

16. 5% dextrose half saline + Half saline 1 L iv c 40 mL/hr

17. Combiflex peri 1100 1.1 L c 40 mL/hr

18. 5% albumin 20 mL/hr

19. Alprostadil (1.47 ug/kg in NS 50 mL) x 12 hr mivs c 4 cc/hr

20. Gabexate (20 mg/kg in NS 50 mL) mivs c 2 cc/hr

21. Heparization nomogram without loading dose (depending on artery state and bleeding tendency)

22. Cefotaxime 2 iv q 8hrs (renal function 에 따라 조절하여야 함)

23. Ampicillin/sulbactam 1.5 g 1A q 6hrs

24. Itraconazole syrup 100 mg PLT Q12

25. Consider Clopidogrel, Warfarin after confirm (POD #5 start)

26. Famotidine 1A + NS 50 mL iv q 12hr

27. Ambroxol 1A ivs q 8hr

28. Diogel 1p PLT HS

29. Octreotide 100q sc q 8 hr

30. PRN) Nifedipine 10 mg SL (If SBP > 160)

31. PRN) Morphine 2 mg iv

32. CBC, e, chemistry, ion Ca, PT/aPTT, S-osm, ABGA, UA c micro, urine (e, osm), chest AP (portable) amylase/lipase

33. CBC, e, BUN/Cr, S-osm/U-osm q 8hr

34. C-peptide, HbA1C, Proinsulin/insulin : Twice a week

35. Immunosuppression

36. POD#1,3,5 Doppler Sono of pancreas

37. Foley remove after checking DTPA and CT angiography
    J-P remove when patient is stable after enough diet

38. Move to general ward depending on patient condition

39. Consult to Infectionist part before discharge and make an appoint at Out patient department

40. CMV 및 bacterial 검사는 kidney transplantation patient에 준하여 검사한다.
    치료 역시 kidney transplantation 환자에 준하여 시행

SUPPLEMENT

Appendix. Intraoperative drugs given during Transplantation

1. Liver transplantation

(*는 필요한 경우 투여하며 수술이 종료되면 남은 Foy, PGE1, Fragmin은 폐
기한다.)

    1) Adult liver transplantation

        (1) Antibiotics: 마취 유도 시 & q 4hr에

        cefotaxim 1 gm IVS (skin test at ward)

        ubacillin 3 gm IVS (skin test at ward)

     * (2) HBsAg (+) recipient: Hepatectomy 직후 & liver out 확인하고
        HB immune globulin 투여한다.

        Hepabig 10,000 U mixed in D5W 200 & IV slowly (100 mL/hr

or 30gtt)

HBcAb (+) donor 경우에도 de novo infection risk 있으므로 투여한다.

Recipient HBeAg (+) or HBV DNA positive인경우에는 20,000 U을 투여한다.

Recipient HBV negative seroconversion 시에는 투여하지 않는다.

(3) Steroid: Hepatic vein anastomosis 종료 후 & 재관류 전에 Solumedrol 500 mg IVS

(4) Simulect: 재관류 후 지혈이 되면(대개 재관류 5분 후에) 20 mg IVS

*(5) Foy, PGE1: LDLT시에만 투여하며, 재관류 후 연결한다.

Foy 1 ampule (50 mg) mixed in D5W 30 mL & IV with 10 mL/hr

PGE1 5 ampule (50 mcg) mixed in D5W 30 mL & IV with 10 mL/hr

2) Pediatric liver transplantation

(1) Antibiotics: 마취 유도 시 & q 4hr에

cefotaxim 25 mg/kg IVS (skin test at ward)

ubacillin 50 mg/kg IVS (skin test at ward)

*(2) HBsAg (+) recipient: Hepatectomy 직후 & liver out 확인하고 HB immunoglobulin 투여한다.

Hepabig 100 U /kg mixed in D5W 20 mL & IV slowly over 3hr

HBcAb (+) donor 경우에도 de novo infection risk 있으므로 투여한다.

(3) Steroid: Hepatic vein anastomosis 종료 후 & 재관류 전에 Solumedrol 20 mg/kg IVS

(4) Foy, PGE1, Fragmin (preparation by GS intern): 재관류 후 연결한다.

Foy 20 mg/kg mixed in D5W 24 mL & IV with 1 mL/hr

PGE1 2 mcg/kg mixed in D5W 24 mL & IV with 2 mL/hr

*Fragmin 50 IU/kg mixed in NS 24 mL & IV with 1 mL/hr

2. Living donor kidney transplantation

〈 Recipient 외과 약 - *basiliximab, rATG 중 어느 약을 투여하는지 반드시 확인한다. 〉

1) Antibiotics: induction 직후에 투여한 후 8시간마다 한 번씩 투여한다.

*2) Simulect (basilixmab) 투여하는 경우 induction 후에 20 mg IV

rATG (1.5 mg/kg) 투여하는 경우 induction 후에 Avil 1ampule IV

〉〉 rATG을 5dw 250 mL mix하여 40 mL/hr IV with Dial-A-Flow & filter

3) 재관류전(graft in직후가 적절):

Solumedrol 500 mg IV, Lasix 40 mg IV, Mannitol (15%) 1 gm / kg (BWt) infusion

3. Deceased donor kidney transplantation

〈 Recipient 외과 약 - *basiliximab, rATG 중 어느 약을 투여하는지 반드시 확인한다. 〉

1) Antibiotics: induction 직후에 투여한 후 8시간마다 한 번씩 투여한다.

*2) Simulect (basilixmab) 투여하는 경우 induction 후에 20 mg IV

*anti-thymocyte globulin (rATG) 투여하는 경우 induction 후에 Avil 1ampule IV 후

rATG (1.5 mg/kg)을 외과에서 갖고 온 수액에 mix하여 12시간 동안 지속 정주.

3) 재관류전(graft in직후가 적절)

(dual kidney 이식 시에는 첫 번째 kidney 재관류 전에 세 가지 약을
다 주고 두 번째 kidney 재관류 전에는 solumedrol과 lasix를 준다.)
Solumedrol 500 mg IV, Lasix 40 mg IV, Mannitol (15%) 1 gm / kg
(BWt) infusion
(소아 KT 외과 약은 외과와 상의한다.)

4. Pancreas Transplantation

Surgery Request

1. Albumin (5%)

   췌장 단독 이식:

   If CVP < 4 mmHg → 2 mL/kg/hr

   < 8 mmHg → 1 mL/kg/hr

   ≥ 8 mmHg → Stop

   신장 동시 이식:

   If CVP < 4 mmHg → 2 mL/kg/hr

   < 10 mmHg → 1 mL/kg/hr

   ≥ 10 mmHg → Stop

2. Antibiotics q 4hr

3. 마취 유도 후 somatostatin 100 mcg 피하 주사한다.

4. anti-thymocyte globulin (ATG) 투여하는 경우 induction 후에 Avil
   1ampule IV 후

   ATG (1.5 mg/kg)을 외과에서 갖고 온 수액에 mix하여 12시간 동안 지
   속 정주

5. 췌장 재관류 전에 solumedrol 500 mg 정주한다.
   (신장 동시 이식 시에는 처음 장기 재관류 전에 투여한다.)

6. 췌장 재관류 후에 Foy, PGE1을 지속 정주한다.

Foy 1 ampule (50 mg) mixed in D5W 30 mL & IV with 10 mL/hr

PGE1 5 ampule (50 mcg) mixed in D5W 30 mL & IV with 10 mL/hr

7. 신장 동시 이식 시에는 Lasix 40 mg 정주하며 mannitol은 투여하지 않는다.

Appendix. Interpretation of Doppler US : Hepatic vasculatures

1. Hepatic artery

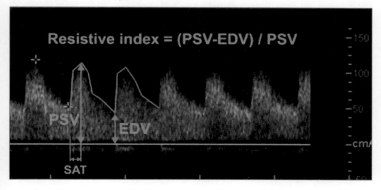

1) Rapid systolic upstroke: SAT (systolic acceleration time) ⟨ 80 ms

2) PSV (Peak systolic velocity): mean-103 cm/s, widely variable

3) Resistive index (RI)= (PSV-EDV)/PSV (normal: 0.55~0.8)EDV↓→ RI↑, PSV↓ or EDV↑→ RI↓

4) Pulsatile low-resistance waveform with a broad systolic peak, antegrade diastolic peak, and spectral broadening

5) Stenosis over 50% is characterized by

   (1) Focal velocity >2 m/sec associated with turbulence

   (2) RI < 0.5

(3) Systolic Acceleration Times (SAT) > 0.8 sec

(4) high-velocity with spectral broadening

(5) Dampened waveform

6) Increased RI: usually resolves with time   cause: allograft edema, long CIT, vessel spasm, etc.

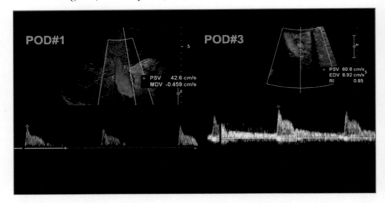

7) Tardus Parvus pattern: delayed SAT with low PAT and low RI

→ Severe stenosis, hepatic artery thrombosis

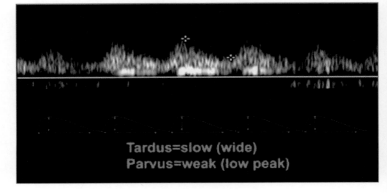

2. Portal vein

1) Antegrade & continuous flow: velocity=20~30 cm/sec

2) No specific difference of velocity and diameter between pre- & post anastomosis site

3) Pulsatility is typically absent

4) Portal vein stenosis: Significant difference in diameter and velocity

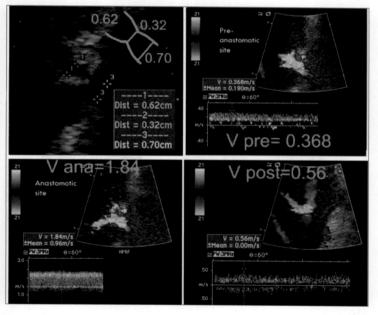

5) Direction of portal flow

    (1) Hepatopetal: flow toward liver

    (2) Hepatofugal: flow away from the liver

    (3) Porto-systemic collateral flow can interfere with the

hepatopetal flow when it is remained with no ligation

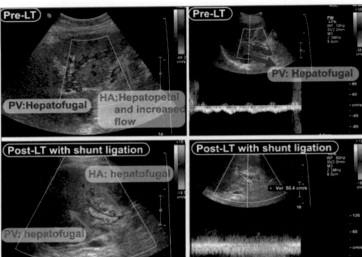

3. Hepatic Vein

1) Triphasic waveform with both respiratory variation and cardiac pulsation

2) Loss of triphasicity does not imply the presence of hepatic venous complication

Appendix. Drug interactions of antimicrobials and immunosuppressants (Sparkes et al., Clin Transplant, 2019,33(9), e13510)

Antimicrobial		Immunosuppressant	Severity	Suggested actions
Macrolides : ↑ Imm levels	Erythromycin	CSA, TAC, SRL, EVR	+++	Avoid/↓ Imm up to 1/2
		Methylprednisolone	++	Utilize prednisone or azithromycin
	Clarithromycin	CSA, TAC, SRL, EVR	+++	Avoid/↓ Imm by 1/2
		Methylprednisolone	++	Utilize prednisone or azithromycin
	Azithromycin	CSA, TAC, SRL, EVR		No adjustmentt
Rifamycins : ↓ Imm levels	Rifampin	CSA, TAC, SRL, EVR	+++	Avoid/↑ Imm 2-fold and monitor
		MMF, MPA	+	Utilize alternate rifamycin if possible
		Prednisone	++	Monitor steroid efficacy, consider dose increase
	Rifabutin	CSA, TAC, SRL, EVR	++	Monitor Imm levels
	Rifapentine	CSA, TAC, SRL, EVR, Prednisone	++	Monitor Imm levels
Aminoglycosides : Nephrotoxicity	Gentamicin, Tobramycin, Amikacin, Streptomycin	CSA, TAC	+++	Avoid/Monitor renal function
Fluoroquinolones	Ciprofloxacin, Ofloxacin, Levofloxacin, Moxifloxacin	CSA, TAC (QTc Prolongation)	++	Monitor QTc and Electrolytes
		Prednisone, MPD (Tendonitis)	++	Monitor
	Ciprofloxacin	MMF, MPA(↓ Imm)	+−	Monitor
Other antibacterials	Nafcillin	CSA, TAC, SRL, EVR	+	↓ Imm levels: monitor
	Quinupristin/ Dalfopristin	CSA, Expected for TAC, SRL, EVR	+++	↑ CSA: monitor
	Chloramphenicol	CSA, Expected for TAC, SRL, EVR	++	↑ Imm Levels: ↓ CSA or TAC by 25%
	Tigecycline	CSA	+−	↑ Tigecycline: Monitor Imm
	Metronidazole Metronidazole	CSA, TAC, SRL, EVR	+−	May ↑ Imm Levels: no adjustment
		MMF, MPA	+	May ↓ Imm levels: Monitor

Other antibacterials	Clindamycin	CSA, TAC, SRL, EVR	+-	May ↓ Imm levels: No adjustment consider monitor levels
	Linezolid	MMF, MPA, AZA, SRL, EVR	++	Myelosuppression: Monitor WBC and platelets
	TMP-SMX TMP-SMX	MMF, MPA, AZA, SRL,EVR	++	Myelosuppression: Monitor WBC, Hct, platelets
		CSA, TAC	++	Nephrotoxicity: renal monitor
Antimalarials : ↓ Imm levels	Artemether/ Lumefantrine	CSA, TAC, SRL, EVR	+	Monitor Imm levels
Antifungals : azoles ↑ Imm levels	Ketoconazole	CSA, TAC, SRL, EVR	+++	Avoid/ ↓ Imm by 1/2
		Methylprednisolone	++	↓ Imm by 1/2
	Voriconazole	CSA, TAC, SRL, EVR	+++	↓ CSA by 1/2, ↓ Tac by 2/3
		Methylprednisolone	+	Monitor
	Itraconazole	CSA, TAC, SRL, EVR	+++	↓ Imm by 1/2, Monitor Imm
		Methylprednisolone	++	↓ Imm by 1/2
	Posaconazole	CSA, TAC, SRL, EVR	+++	↓ CSA by 1/4, ↓ Tac by 2/3
		Methylprednisolone	+	Monitor
	Isavuconazole	CSA, TAC, SRL, EVR	++	Monitor Imm levels
		MMF, MPA	+-	Monitor for MMF, MPA ADE's
	Fluconazole	CSA, TAC, SRL, EVR	++	Dose dependent
	Clotrimazole	CSA, TAC, SRL, EVR	++	Monitor Imm Levels
Antifungals: Echinocandins	Caspofungin	CSA	++	↑ Caspofungin levels: monitor LFT
		TAC	+-	May ↓ TAC levels: no adjustment
	Micafungin	CSA	++	↓ CSA levels: monitor imm
		SRL	+	↑ SRL levels: monitor imm
	Anidulafungin	CSA	+	↑ Anidulafungin: none
Antifungals: Polyenes	Amphotericin B	CSA, TAC (renal toxicity)	++	Monitor renal function, Utilize lipid-based products if appropriate
Other antifungals	Flucytosine	MMF, MPA, AZA, SRL,EVR	++	Myelosuppression: Monitor WBC, hematocrit, platelets

Antivirals (non-HIV and non-HCV)	Acyclovir	MMF, MPA	+-	↑ Acyclovir in presence of renal impairment: None
	IV acyclovir	CSA, TAC (nephrotoxic)	+++	Monitor renal function
	Ganciclovir, Valganciclovir	MMF, MPA, AZA, SRL, EVR	++	Myelosuppression: Monitor WBC
	Ribavirin	AZA (Accumulation of 6-methylthioinosine and myelotoxicity)	+++	Avoid
	Foscarnet	CSA, TAC(nephrotoxic, ↓ Ca, ↓ Mg)	+++	Avoid/Monitor renal function, Ca, Mg
	Cidofovir	CSA, TAC (nephrotoxic)	+++	Avoid/Monitor renal functiont
	Leflunomide	MMF, MPA, AZA (myelosuppression)	+++	Avoid/Monitor WBC, hematocrit and platelets
	Letermovir	CSA (↑ CSA, ↑ Letermovir)	+++	Decrease Letermovir to 240 mg once daily in combination with CSA, Monitor Imm levels
		TAC (↑ TAC)	+++	Monitor Imm levels
		SRL, EVR (↑ SRL)	+++	Monitor Imm levels
Antiretroviral agents: Protease inhibitors ↑ Imm levels Antiretroviral agents: Protease inhibitors ↑ Imm levels	Atazanavir, Darunavir, Fosamprenavir, Indinavir, Lopinavir/ ritonavir, Nelfinavir, Ritonavir, Saquinavir, Tipranavir/ ritonavir	CSA, TAC, SRL, EVR	+++	Avoid if possible. CSA 25-50 mg daily TAC 1 mg once or twice a week SRL 1 mg once or twice a week. Monitor Imm levels
		Prednisone	++	Monitor for symptoms of Cushing's syndrome

Antiretroviral agents: Cytochrome P450 inhibitor	Cobicistat	CSA, TAC, SRL, EVR	+++	↑ Imm levels Avoid if possible TAC 0.5-1.5 mg once or twice a week Monitor Imm Levels
Antiretroviral agents: Non-nucleoside reverse transcriptase inhibitors	Efavirenz	CSA, TAC, SRL, EVR	++	↓ Imm levels: monitor imm
	Nevirapine, Etravirine	CSA, TAC, SRL, EVR	+-	May ↓ Imm levels: monitor imm
	Delavirdine	CSA, TAC, SRL, EVR	++	↑ Imm levels: monitor imm
Antiretroviral agents: Nucleoside reverse transcriptase inhibitors	Tenofovir disoproxil fumarate	CSA, TAC (nephrotoxicity)	++	Monitor, consider tenofovir alafenamide
	Stavudine, Zidovudine	MMF/MPA (in vitro antagonism)	+-	None
Antiretroviral agents: HCV DAA	Paritaprevir/ ritonavir/ ombitasvir + dasabuvir (PrOD)	CSA (5.8-fold ↑ in CSA AUC)	+++ +++	Use 1/5 CSA, monitor CSA levels
		TAC (57-fold ↑ in TAC AUC)	+++ +++	Avoid
		SRL (38-fold ↑ in SRL AUC)		
		EVR (27-fold ↑ in EVR AUC)		
	Elbasvir/ grazoprevir (EBR/GZR)	CSA (15-fold ↑ in GZR AUC and 2-fold ↑ in EBR AUC)	+++	Avoid
		TAC (43% ↑ in TAC AUC)	++	Monitor TAC levels
		SRL,EVR (↑ Imm)	+	Monitor Imm levels
	Sofosbuvir/ velpatasvir (SOF/VEL)	CSA, TAC, SRL, EVR (↑ Imm)	+	Monitor Imm levels
	Sofosbuvir/ velpatasvir/ voxilaprevir (SOF/ VEL/ VOX)	CSA (9.4-fold ↑ in VOX AUC)	+++	Avoid, VOX and CSA combination not recommended
		TAC, SRL, EVR (↑ Imm)	+	Monitor Imm levels

Antiretroviral agents: HCV DAA	Glecaprevir/ pibrentasvir (GLE/PIB)	CSA (5-fold ↑ in GLE AUC with higher doses (400 mg) of CSA 5-fold ↑ in PIB AUC with higher doses of CSA)	+++	Not recommended in patients requiring stable CSA doses > 100 mg/day
		TAC (1.45-fold ↑ in TAC AUC)	+	Monitor Imm levels
		SRL, EVR (↑ Imm)	+	Monitor Imm levels
	Simeprevir (SMP)	CSA (5.8-fold ↑ in Simeprevir with CSA)	+++	Avoid, Simeprevir and CSA combination not recommended
		TAC (1.85-fold ↑ in Simeprevir exposure, ↓ TAC)	+	Monitor TAC levels
		SRL, EVR (Potential ↑ or ↓ in Imm levels)	+	Monitor Imm levels

Appendix. Blood glucose control for NPO patients

A. Modified Alberti' s regimen

* Indication: HbA1c < 7%, preoperative BST constantly maintained <180 mg/dL with previous medication

1. Initiation: RI 15 U + 20 mEq KCl in 1000 mL 5% DW, 100 mL/hr (protocol A)

   or RI 30 U + 2 0mEq KCl in 1000 mL 10% DW, 100 mL/hr (protocol B)

   1) BST q 2hr (q 1hr if necessary), electrolyte q 12h since overnight fasting

   2) 5% or 10% DW 1000 mL + KCl 20 mEq/L (2M KCl로 10 mL) with 100 mL/h mivIf K < 4 mEq/L, increase KCl to 40 mEq/L (2M KCl로 20 mL)If 4 < K < 5 mEq/L, continue to 20 mEq/L (2M KCl로 10 mL)If K > 5 mEq/L, delete KCl

2. Target BST: 140-180 mg/dl

Plasma glucose (mg/dL)	Insulin volume (U/L)	
	Protocol A	Protocol B
<80	5 ↓	10 ↓
<120	3 ↓	5 ↓
120-180	No change	
>180	3 ↑ (if BST is declining, do not increase)	5 ↑ (if BST is declining, do not increase)
>270	5 ↑ (if BST is declining, do not increase)	10 ↑ (if BST is declining, do not increase)

B. Computerized IV insulin protocol

* Indication: HbA1c > 8% or preoperative BST > 180 mg/dL despite previous medication

1. Prepration: 0.9% NaCl 2 mL + regular insulin (RI) 1 unit (rate can be altered by 0.5 U/hr)

2. Pretreatment: To prevent adherence of insulin to IV line, fill up the line with insulin mixed saline 20 mL.

3. Target BST: 140-180 mg/dL

4. Initiation: Round off base BST/100 (if base BST is 270 mg/dL, 270/100=2.7 ⇨ 3 U/hr), then it is the initial infusion rate

5. When BST<70, stop insulin. Inject 50% DW 50 mL and BST q 15min till BST≥110. 1 hr later, if BST≥140, decrease 2△ and restart the insulin.

6. Infusion rate adjustment protocol

BST<100	100≤BST<140	140≤BST<180	180≤BST<260	260≤BST	Guideline
			40≤ ΔBS*	0≤ ΔBS	Increase 2△
		20≤ ΔBS	0≤ ΔBS<40	-40≤ ΔBS<0	Increase 1△
10≤ ΔBS	0≤ ΔBS	-20≤ ΔBS<20	-40≤ ΔBS<0	-80≤ ΔBS<-40	No change

-10≤⊿BS<10	-20≤⊿BS<0	-40≤⊿BS<-20	-80≤⊿BS<-40	-120≤⊿BS<-80	Decrease 1△
⊿BS<-10	⊿BS<-20	⊿BS<-40	⊿BS<-80	⊿BS<-120	Stop for 2 hrs. If BST≤140, decrease 2△ then restart

* ⊿BS; Blood sugar change per hour

Infusion Rate (U/hr)	△ = Rate change (U/hr)	2△ = Rate change (U/hr)
RI < 3	0.5	1
3≤ RI <6	1	2
6 ≤ RI < 10	1.5	3
10 ≤ RI < 15	2	4

Appendix. Heparinization nomogram

- Normal saline 500 mL + Heparin 25000 unit (50 unit/mL)

- Target apt 60~85 sec

- Initial start : maintain IV 12 unit/kg/hr

- aPTT check : heparin 시작 6시간 후, 그 후는 nomogram에 따라 check 후 notify

aPTT (sec)	Bolus or hold	Rate change	aPTT re-check
aPTT < 50	Bolus 3000U ivs	Increase by 3 cc/hr,	after 6hr
50 ≤ aPTT < 60sec	-	Increase by 2 cc/hr	after 6hr
60 ≤ aPTT < 86sec	-	No change	next AM
86 ≤ aPTT < 96sec	-	Decrease by -1 cc/hr	next AM
96 ≤ aPTT < 120sec	Hold for 30min	Decrease by -2 cc/hr	after 6hr
aPTT ≥ 120	Hold for 60min	Decrease by -3 cc/hr	after 6hr

Appendix . Nutrition protocol for LT patients
1. 원칙

- 모든 LT 환자는 Parenteral Nutrition (PN)보다 Enteral Nutrition (EN) 을 우선시.
- EN 공급 중이나 목표열량의 60% 이상 공급이 어려운 경우 supplementary PN 고려

2. =Indication and Timing

- EN: 이식 전] 정상 식이 진행이 목표열량의 50% 미만 섭취가 1주 이상 지속된 환자 중 enteral route를 통한 feeding이 가능한 모든 환자.
  이식 후] 기저 질환 Child B or C인 환자 중 enteral route feeding 가능 환자.
  - 환자의 영양상태와 관계 없이 24시간 이내에 시작
  - 장운동의 근거(Stool, Flatus, Bowel sound)는 필요하지는 않음
- PN: 3일 이내에 oral diet가 불가능할 것으로 판단되는 환자 중 enteral route를 통한 feeding이 불가능한 모든 환자.
  - 환자가 malnutrition이 동반된 경우는 EN와 마찬가지로 24-48시간 이내에 시작
  - 환자가 well nourished patient 일 경우라면 정상 식이 진행해서 목표 열량의 50%이상 도달하지 못할 때
- 혈역학적으로 안정적이며 Fluid Resuscitation이 완료된 상태여야 함.
  - "혈역학적 안정"이란 Vasopressor가 지속적으로 tapering되거나 Low dose 유지 상태로 주치의의 판단으로 결정
  - ⇨ Indication이 되어 치료 시작시 영양지원팀(NST, Nutrition Support Team) 협진의뢰

3. Selection of Route

- EN

  - Feeding 시작 시 특별한 사유가 없는 이상 Enteral Feeding Tube 를 이용한 Nasogastric Feeding을 우선 시행함

    - ◆ Feeding tube insertion 시 반드시 X-ray로 위치 확인 후 공급 시작

  - 아래와 같은 경우 Nasojejunal (post-pyloric) Feeding 사용

    - ◆ Gastric Feeding에 지속적인 Intolerance 가 있을 경우

    - ⇨ Vomiting, Regurgitation, Gastric emptying에 장애가 있을 경우

    - ◆ Aspiration의 위험성이 높은 경우

    - ⇨ Nasojejunal Feeding Tube Insertion은 우선적으로 Endoscopic Guide로 시행함.

      (IM1 장동경 또는 김은란 교수님 의뢰, 처방코드 RA3408)

      내시경이 불가능할 경우 영상의학과에 의뢰하여 투시조영으로 시행

  - 6주 이상 지속 시 또는 6주 이상으로 예상되는 경우(long-term EN) ⇨ Percutaneous endoscopic gastrostomy (PEG 경피적 위루 설치술), Gastrostomy, Transgastric jejunostomy, Surgical jejunostomy 고려.

- PN

  - low osmolarity (<850 mOsmol/L)의 PN 제제를 사용할 경우에는 peripheral access

  - Low osmolarity PN만으로 환자의 요구량을 만족하지 못하는 경우, 2주이상 장기간 PN이 필요한 경우는 central access

  - central access가 지속적으로 필요하며 hemodynamic하게 stable

한 경우는 PICC insertion을 고려

4. Administration

- Goal
  - 이식 전: 30-35 kcal/kg/day
  - 이식 후: Acute phase: 20-25 kcal/kg/day
    Recovery Phase 30-35 kcal/kg/day
    ⇨ 칼로리 계산하는 Body Weight 산정
    - Ideal BW < Actual BW 일 경우 Ideal BW 사용
    - Actual BW < Ideal BW 일 경우 Actual BW 사용
      * [BMI>30]일 경우 두 값 사이의 중간 값 또는 적은 쪽 1/4 값을 사용
        - 항상 overfeeding을 주의해야 함.
- Method, Dose, Advancing
  - EN
    - 모든 환자에서 feeding 전용 pump를 이용한 continuous Feeding 시행
    - 시작 시 Full Strength Formula로 시작함.
    - 20~30 cc/hr로 시작, 24시간 연속 투여(FK506 복용 시 20hr/day로 변경)
    - GI tolerance가 괜찮은 경우 목표량까지 8시간 마다 10 cc/hr 증량
    - 목표량에 도달한 경우 총량으로 투여로 처방(예 60 cc/hr ⇨ 1500 cc/day)
    - 환자의 상태가 안정적인 경우 Intermittent Feeding 변경을 고려
  - PN

- ◆ 16~20 kcal/kg/day로 시작
- ◆ 환자 상태를 관찰 하면서 2~3일 동안 20~25 kcal/kg/day으로 증량
- ◆ 환자 상태가 안정화되면 목표 열량을 다시 산정하여 증량을 고려
- ● 장기간 영양공급을 받지 못했던 환자의 경우 refeeding syndrome에 주의
- ⇨ Potassium, magnesium, phosphate replace 후 시작
- ⇨ 더 적은 칼로리로(통상, 10% dextrose) 시작하여 더 느린 속도로 증량

- ■ Macronutrients 결정
  - ◆ Amino acid: 0.8~2.5 g/kg/day
  - ● 이식 후 기본적으로 1.3-1.5 g/kg/day 정도를 권고
  - ● PN 시작 첫 날부터 amino acid의 목표량을 모두 투여할 수 있음
  - ● Stress, 신기능이나 간기능에 따라 공급량을 조절
  - ● Normal renal function

Mild stress	0.8~1.2 g/kg/d
Moderate stress	1.3~1.5 g/kg/d
Severe stress	1.5~2.0 g/kg/d

  - ◆ Lipid: 1 g/Kg/Day 또는 전체 칼로리의 20-30% 공급
  - ● 일반적으로 high soybean oil lipid는 권고하지 않음
  - ● 현재는 soybean이 적고 fish oil이 들어 있는 SMOF lipid(원내 코드: XSMOF1, 20 g/100 mL)를 우선 고려
  - ◆ Carbohydrate: amino acid, lipid로 결정된 칼로리의 나머지를 공급

- Minimal amount는 2 g/kg/day
- 대략 3 ~ 6 g/kg/day

5. Supplementary PN

- EN만으로 목표 칼로리에 도달하지 못할 경우 부족한 칼로리를 PN으로 공급
- Supplementary PN 시작 시점
  - Well nourished 환자에서는 EN만으로 7일째까지 100% 도달하지 못하였을 경우 부족한 칼로리만큼 시작을 권고 ⇨ 7일 이후에는 목표 칼로리의 100%를 반드시 공급해야 함.
  - Moderate degree 이상의 malnutrition이 있는 경우에는 3-4일째부터 부족한 칼로리를 PN으로 보충하는 early supplement PN을 고려

6. Monitoring

- GI tolerance
  - Stool의 양상 관찰: frequency, volume, consistency, color
  - Abdominal distension 발생 유무 관찰.
  - Vomiting, aspiration 유무 관찰
  - 주 1-2회 abdomen supine x-ray 확인(EN 종료시까지)
    ⇨ feeding tube location, ileus 확인
  - Gastric residual check
    - Gastric feeding시 4hr 마다 check
    - Check후 Gastric Contents는 다시 주입(GRV 250cc이상 시 재주입 하지 않음)
    - gastric residual volume threshold
      - 250cc 이상일 경우 급식 중단 후 원인에 대한 Evaluation 시행

- 특별한 이유 없이 지속적으로 250cc 이상일 경우 prokinetics 고려
  - IV 제제 : Metoclopramide (XMETO 1 Amp (10 mg)) q 8hr, 1일 최대량-3 Amp ⇨ 5일 이내 사용을 권고함. 5일 후에도 지속될 경우 oral 제제 고려
  - Oral 제제 : Mosapride (MOSA 1정(5 mg) TID)
  - Prokinetics table 참고
- Prokinetics 투여 후에도 지속적으로 250 cc 이상일 경우 Gastric Emptying 장애로 판단하고 바로 Nasojejunal Feeding을 고려.
- Intermittent feeding 시 Feeding 시작 직전 GRV가 250 cc 이상일 경우 4hrs 이후 re-check
- Tube Flushing
  - ◆ Continuous Feeding시 4시간마다 또는 Residual Check 후 최소 30 cc 이상(회신서 참조)의 물을 Flushing함.
  - ◆ Sterile Water(멸균 증류수-처방코드 XWL) 및 생리식염수(Normal Saline) 사용 가능 ⇨ 정수기 및 기타 모든 음료 제한
- Nutritional Status
  - ◆ Check Daily Body Weight
  - ◆ 환자가 안정화 때까지, ionized Ca, Mg, P 포함한 전해질과 혈당을 매일 확인
  - ◆ Prealbumin level check – EN start 전, 매주 월요일
  - ◆ Inadequate Nutritional supply가 의심되는 경우 Nitrogen balance 측정
    - Protein, 24hr Urine, 검사코드 BL 3221
    - GFR <50일 경우 의미 없음

◆ 1개월 이상 PN을 지속할 경우 Zinc, Selenium의 혈중 농도를 확인

◆ TPN을 하는 경우 주 1회 Vitamin K를 공급

7. Formula Selection

- EN
  - Start Formula: Fiber-free RTH (Ready to hanging)로 시작
    - ◆ 경구약 처방 Formula: Encover (ENCO4-S (400 mL))
    - ◆ 뉴케어300 RTH, 메디웰 화이버리스 RTH, 케어웰인텐시브 RTH
  - Secondary modification: 환자 상태에 따라 NST와 진료과가 상의 하여 조정

    (EN formula table 참고)

- PN
  - 환자 상태, 영양 요구량에 맞는 상품형 PN을 사용
  - 다음의 경우 NST에 의뢰하여 약제부에서 조제한 PN을 투여
    - 특별한 질환을 동반한 경우
    - 전해질 불균형이 발생한 경우
    - 영양 요구량이 상품형 PN과 맞지 않는 경우
    - ICU 사용이 권고되는 상품형 PN
      - ◆ 말초정맥용
      - ◆ XOLIM-P (700 kcal/1,000 mL, 25 g amino acid, 30 g lipid = 올리브유:대두유=80%:20%)
      - ◆ XSKABP (1,006 kcal/1,448 mL, 46 g amino acid, 41 g lipid = XSMOF)
      - ◆ 중심정맥용
      - ◆ XWINUF (1,184 kcal/1,085 mL, 55 g amino acid, 41 g

= XSMOF)

- ◆ XWIN14 (1,566 kcal/1,250 mL, 70 g amino acid, 50 g
  = XSMOF)

- ◆ XSKAB20 (2,154 kcal/1,970 mL, 100 g amino acid, 75 g
  = XSMOF)

- ◆ 환자 상태에 따라 상기의 제품 외에도 다른 상품형 PN 사용 가능

8. Complications

- ● Aspiration 예방
  - ■ Feeding 시 30~45도의 Head Elevation Position
  - ■ Vomiting 발생 시 Tube Function을 Check하고 Infusion Rate를 낮춤.
  - ■ Delayed Gastric Emptying이 의심될 경우
    - ● Narcotic mediation 중단 및 감량, 고려,
    - ● Low Fat or Isotonic Formula 변경 고려
    - ● Feeding Rate를 20~25 cc/hr로 감량 고려
    - ● Prokinetics 사용 고려
- ● Diarrhea
  - ■ 정의(ASPEN core curriculum 2012): 500 mL/day 이상 또는 연속 2일 이상 하루 3회 이상일 경우
  - ■ 원인 규명이 우선
    - ◆ Infectious vs Osmotic vs Intolerance
    - ◆ eg: Medications, Abdominal Exam, Fecal Leukocytes, Quantification of stool, Stool culture, Serum electrolyte, Review of medication, C.difficile toxin assay

- 원인에 대한 처치를 시행.
- 심할 경우 주입 속도를 줄이고 수용성 섬유소(soluble fiber) 함유 영양액, Low FODMAP formula으로 변경.
- Infectious diarrhea가 아니면서 지속될 경우 Antidiarrheal Agent 적용을 검토.
- Probiotics 고려 ⇨ 람노스과립® (RHAM-P, 2포(2 g) BID, 1일 최대량-8포(8 g)
- loperamide oxide (LOPEO, 1일1정(2 mg) 4회, 1일 최대량 8정 (16 mg))
- Smectite (SMEC-K , 1 팩 TID)
    ⇨ intermittent feeding 시 공복에 투여
    ⇨ continuous feeding 시 금지(약효발현↓ 영양흡수↓)
- Constipation
  - Defecation이 주 2회 이하일 경우 주의
  - Fecal Impaction이 있을 때 Fiber-free 영양액을 사용 & 수분공급 증가
  - 지속될 경우 Stool Softner나 Water Bolus 사용을 고려.
    - Lactulose syrup (LACTE-S, 10~45 mL QD 아침) (주의)고혈당 환자
    - 둘코락스 좌약(BISA-Y, Bisacodyl 1 개 (10 mg))
    - Magnesium oxide (MGO, 1 정(500 mg) BID~QID) : (주의) 신장애 환자
- Hyperglycemia
  - BST 140~180 mg/dl 목표
  - 각 중환자실에 따른 RI infusion scale 적용
  - DM formula 사용

● VAP 예방

■ 기계환기 중인 환자에게는 금기증이 없는 한 probiotics를 투여한
다.

⇨ 람노스과립® (RHAM-P, 2포(2 g) BID, 1일 최대량-8포(8 g))

9. Nutrition therapy의 종료

● 충분한 oral intake가 가능한 경우

● SFD 또는 SBD 진행 후 평가하여 충분한 경우 EN 중단(영양요구량의
70% 이상 섭취)

● PN을 공급 하는 중에도 매일 EN의 가능성에 대하여 고려

● EN을 시작하게 될 경우 공급량에 맞게 PN 칼로리를 감량
(overfeeding 주의)

Table 1. EN formula

구분	영양액	특성
Fiber-free (% of protein)	뉴케어300RTH(16%), 뉴케어300 메디웰화이버리스RTH (18%) 케어웰인텐시브 RTH (20%) Encover(18%)	Diarrhea 주의
Standard formulas	뉴케어300 그린비아TF 메디푸드(powder)	Intact protein, CHO, fat 함유

Closed system	뉴케어300RTH 뉴케어화이버RTH 뉴케어당뇨 RTH 메디웰화이버리스 RTH 메디웰화이버RTH 메디웰당뇨 RTH Encover Harmonilan	RTH (Ready-to-hanging) formula
Fiber-containing	뉴케어화이버 뉴케어화이버RTH 메디웰화이버 메디웰화이버RTH 그린비아장솔루션 그린비아화이버 Harmonilan	Stool consistency 조절 가능
Low FODMAP	그린비아 장솔루션	FODMAP: fermentable oligosaccharides, disaccharides and monosaccharides and polyols (Abdominal distension, cramping, diarrhea 완화에 도움)
High protein	그린비아HP (High Protein)	Protein 비율 25%
Hyperglycemia	메디웰당뇨RTH 메디웰DM 뉴케어당뇨RTH 뉴케어DM 그린비아DM	Carbohydrates 함량 낮으며 fiber 함유함
Azotemia	그린비아RD(비투석제형) 그린비아RD plus(투석제형)	Low to moderate protein Na, K, P, Mg 함량 낮음 Calorie density: 2.0 kcal/mL
Concentrated Formula	메디웰프로틴1.5	1.5배 농축 (1000 mL=1500 kcal)
Low Fat for Chyle Leaks	병원제조 저지방	4.4 g LCT/1000kcal, MCT oil 12.3 g : LCT 4.4 g *Multivitamin & mineral, trace elements 병행 보충 필요

Table 2. Prokinetics

성분	Mosapride	Metoclopramide	Levosulpiride	Itopride	Domperidone	Motiliton®
구조		benzamide			benzimidazole	
약리 기전	• 5-HT4 agonist	• Dopamine D2 receptor antagonist • 5-HT4 receptor facilitation of acetycholine release from enteric nerves • 5-HT3 receptor antagonist	• Dopamine D2 receptor antagonist	• Dopamine D2 receptor antagonist	• Peripheral Dopamine D2 receptor antagonist	• 5-HT4 agonist • Dopamine D2 receptor antagonist
특징	• Enhances upper GI motor activity with minimal or no effect on lower GI motor activity (Controversial) • No significant D2-receptor antagonism, • Lower CNS adverse effects (extrapyramidal symptoms, depression) • No statistically significant impact on cardiac function • Hepatic metabolism via CYP 3A4 • 한국,중국,일본 등 판매 • Not in USA	• ADR :~ 30% Drowsiness, fatigue, agitation, sleep disturbance • ADR: ~16% Extrapyramidal symptoms • EMA (2013.08) :최대 5일간 사용권고 • 식약처(2013.10) :최대치료기간 5일 및 최대 권장용량 0.5 mg/kg/day or 30 mg/day 로 사용제한 • [U.S. Boxed Warning]: May cause tardive dyskinesia, which is often irreversible; duration of treatment and total cumulative dose are associated with an increased risk.	• BBB 일부통과 • ADR : Depression, somatoform disorders, schizophrenia • GI disorders (functional dyspepsia, irritable bowel syndrome, diabetic gastrocholecystoparesis) and emesis prophylaxis in patients with cancer • Not in USA	• BBB 약 1/7 통과 • 우리나라, 체코, 일본, 말레시아, 필리핀, 타이 등 판매 • Not in USA	• Not cross BBB • Hepatic metabolism via CYP 3A4 • Canadian Boxed warning: increased risk of ventricular arrhythmias or sudden cardiac death, particularly with doses >30 mg or patients >60 yr	• Metabolism and excretion: liver

[LT W/U 시 Nutrition Algorithm]

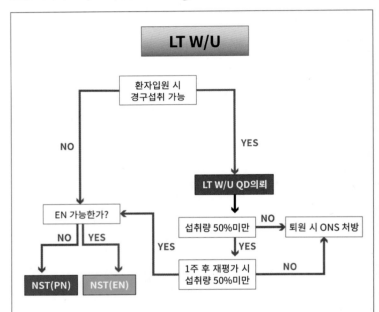

LT W/U 환자 중 입원시점에서

- 경구섭취 불가능한 환자의 경우 EN/PN 고려
- 경구섭취 가능한 환자의 경우 LT W/U 진행하여 식사량 50% 미만으로 섭취 시 1주 후 재평가를 통해 식사섭취 지속적으로 저하된 상태일 경우, EN/PN 고려
- 식사섭취 양호한 환자의 경우 퇴원 시 ONS 처방으로 LT 전까지 영양상태 유지

[LT Nutrition Algorithm]

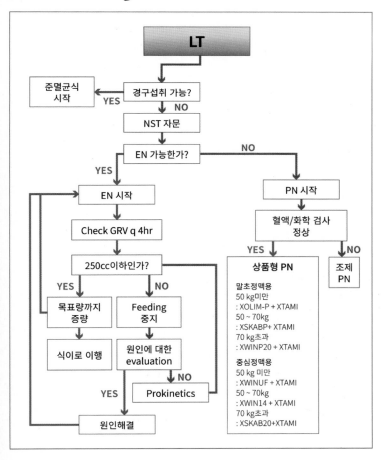

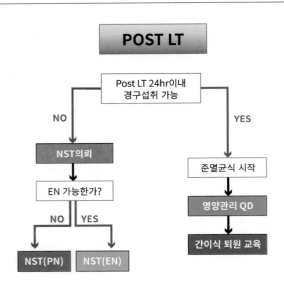

Post LT 환자 중 24hr이내

- 경구섭취 불가능한 환자의 경우 early EN/PN 고려
- 이식전 Child B or C인 환자의 경우 early EN 고려
- 경구섭취 가능한 환자의 경우 SOW → 준멸균식(SFD→ SBD→ NRD)시작
- 준멸균식 식사 시 준멸균식 관련 영양교육 [영양관리] QD 의뢰
- 퇴원 전 [간이식 퇴원교육] QD의뢰